# THE THYROID PATIENT'S MANUAL

## From Hypothyroidism to Good Health Using T4, NDT, T3 or T4/T3 Thyroid Treatments

## PAUL ROBINSON

The information provided in The Thyroid Patient's Manual is for educational purposes only. This book is not intended to replace the care by a qualified, licensed and competent medical professional. Care by a medical professional may be necessary to meet the unique needs of an individual patient. The author and publisher are clear that this book does not in <u>any</u> way represent the practice of medicine.

The author, publisher and others involved in the production and publication of this book do <u>not</u> recommend that readers alter their treatment that has been created for them by their own doctor or other health care professionals without individualised and clear guidance from these health care professionals.

Neither the author, publisher, nor any medical or health practitioners or researchers mentioned, nor any other parties involved in the preparation or publication of this book warrant that the information contained in this book is indicated, applicable, effective or safe in any individual case.

The author, publisher and others involved in the preparation or publication of this book disclaims any liability resulting directly or indirectly from the use of the information contained in this book. A qualified doctor should supervise in all matters relevant to physical or mental health.

Every effort has been made to make this book as complete and accurate as possible. However, there may be mistakes, both typographical and in content. Furthermore, this book contains information that is current only up to the date of publishing.

First published by Elephant in the Room Books 2018

ISBN: 978-0-9570993-3-3

To all thyroid patients, who continue to struggle to get the thyroid hormone treatment that they need in order to fully recover their health. It ought not to be this difficult!

# Acknowledgements

My grateful thanks to the kind-hearted people who reviewed the draft version of this book: Professor Rudolf Hoermann, Erin Lembke, Dr. Henry Lindner, Paul R Lundy, Helen Macdonald, Lynn McGovern, Louise Roberts, Akinyi Shapiro, Darin Strauss, Christel Van Gelder, and Michelle Weiler.

My special thanks to **Professor Rudolf Hoermann** and to **Dr. Henry Lindner**, who both gave so generously of their time to ensure the accuracy of this book and make it a practical manual for thyroid patients. My thanks to **Michelle Weiler**, who helped me with many of the ranges and treatment options in Chapter 21, and to **Lynn McGovern** for her contributions to Chapters 11 and 20.

Thanks also to Michael Lavelle for producing the diagram describing 'Our Energy System'.

I believe *The Thyroid Patient's Manual* will be a valuable, well-used tool over the coming years. I hope that many more thyroid patients will regain their health as a result of reading this book. Thank you all!

# Contents

# Chapter 1

## Introduction

This will be my third book dealing with hypothyroidism. I now have over 30 years of personal knowledge of this condition and over 10 years experience of supporting thyroid patients. My first two books *Recovering with T3* and *The CT3M Handbook* are still considered to be the go-to books for people requiring T3 thyroid hormone treatment.

My first books focused solely on the safe and effective use of T3 (Liothyronine). However, this book is far more general. It is a manual to help people understand thyroid issues, reach a diagnosis and prepare for thyroid treatment. It can also help those who are already on a thyroid treatment that is not working well. It will discuss all the different thyroid medications and provide information on their use and dosage management.

I have written this book using language and terms that most of you should relate to and understand. It is also short, practical, and as easy to read as I could make it, given that some topics are complex by their very nature. It will provide a great resource for people who are trying to understand and fix their hypothyroidism.

*This book covers all thyroid hormone treatment options including T4 (Levothyroxine), NDT (natural desiccated thyroid), T3 and the T4/T3 combination.* After some basic background, it describes a simple series of steps that will help you move through diagnosis, to finding the right treatment. It also helps you to deal with all the common problems that might get in the way. I have tried to keep it at a level that anyone can cope with. However, there are a few sections that were inevitably harder to keep simple. I have done my best to limit the number of these.

I am writing this book because I strongly believe that when people are unwell, and perhaps not thinking as clearly as they used to, there is a need for a very clear, concise manual that covers the essentials, and in the right sequence that people need, in order to get well. I have deliberately kept it brief, but have directed people to other resources and books for more detail. The resources include a few research study references that may be useful when dealing with doctors.

There ought not to be a need for this book at all. However, at this point in time, we require a new paradigm of thyroid hormone diagnosis and treatment to be developed. This new paradigm needs to be in the hands of doctors and endocrinologists. It will take time for this to occur - many years I expect. In the meantime, patients need useful tools like this book to help them through an often-bumpy journey to retrieve their health.

## Who is this book aimed at?

This book is meant to help anyone who suspects that they might have hypothyroidism, or someone who has recently been diagnosed with it. It is also aimed at thyroid patients whose treatment no longer seems to work.

Note: I am **not** going to deal with **hyper**thyroidism (too much thyroid hormone). I am strictly going to focus on the topic of **hypo**thyroidism (low levels or low-effect of thyroid hormones). However, once hyperthyroidism is treated, it often turns into hypothyroidism; in this case, this book will be helpful.

In order to keep things short, relatively simple and easy to read, I have only included essential information. However, I will include links and references when needed. I am not going to provide references for every single assertion that I make. Everything I write I believe to be true. However, my goal is to make the book a very practical manual for thyroid patients, so simplicity and conciseness are essential.

Let me be very clear; this is a patient-to-patient manual and is based on my own experience and the experience of thousands of other people that I have worked with over the past 10 years. It is also rooted in recent thyroid research. It will include views that are likely to be quite different to what you may hear from your own doctor and possibly other patients. I have no intention of being consistent with current medical practices if I believe that they are wrong - and many of them are very wrong! I have also no intention of adhering to views that are often expressed on the Internet if they are wrong.

The book provides background information and guidelines on tests and treatment approaches. It provides reference ranges and typical dosages for replacement of vitamins, minerals and hormones. However, it should not be viewed as a cookbook where you need exactly so much of each ingredient - and no more or less. The guidelines are there for every individual to work through on their own and with their doctor. We are not all the same, and adjustments need to be made in every individual case.

## Overall layout of the book

The book will begin with several chapters that explain how the thyroid gland and thyroid hormones fit into a larger system. When this system works well, it gives us the energy to live our lives. Having a basic grasp of this will help you to understand the relationships between the thyroid gland, its hormones and other hormones produced by our endocrine system.

After the basics are discussed, we will dive straight into understanding hypothyroidism, looking at symptoms and interpreting laboratory test results. All the various thyroid hormone treatments will be explained, with enough detail that you will understand how they are used and what to look out for.

There are four chapters that focus on each of the main thyroid hormone treatments. Each chapter stands alone so that you can focus on the therapy that is most relevant to you at any given time. Hence, there is a great deal of similarity in the structure, and in some of the content in these chapters. This was a deliberate choice. Although it might appear as repetition to some of you, it does allow each of these thyroid medication chapters to be complete enough to help you understand that particular treatment.

Many problems can either stop thyroid treatment from working or masquerade as low thyroid hormone symptoms. I will therefore go through as many of these issues as I can. I will go about doing this in the order that you should consider investigating and dealing with them. Some of these problems need attention immediately in the journey to get well, as they are common and will undermine progress.

Less common issues will also be discussed (so you have this information should you need it). The book will then wrap up with material that does not fit nicely in any of the other chapters.

## Get in the driver's seat and gain some control of your health

This is something that I believe everyone should do, whether they have hypothyroidism or any other health problems. When you understand your health issues, and treatments, far more effective discussions can take place with your doctors. This is, of course, only as long as the doctors are open minded enough to allow you to do so.

Getting in the driver's seat does not mean that someone can manage without a doctor. It just means that we all own our own bodies and should always feel responsible for our own health. It means having enough information to understand your illness and be able to discuss it with your doctor. Being able to ask knowledgeably about test results and treatment options is a good thing. If results look low to you, based on what you know, you ought to be able to talk about them with some confidence to your doctor. If you continue to remain ill, and you think the treatment is not being managed properly, knowing enough to recognise this could mean the difference between a swift recovery and a dreadfully long and drawn out one. In the worst case, if treatment is not going well, and you understand enough to realise why, you will be able to consider finding a better physician.

I do not believe that this book can in any way replace the relationship between a patient and their doctor. However, it ought to give you enough knowledge that you have some control and influence in discussions with your doctor. The consequence of this should be a much faster recovery.

*The above is what I mean throughout the book when I talk about being in the driver's seat.*

## Be prepared

When someone is first diagnosed with hypothyroidism they often think that their doctor will give them a tablet to take each day and that they will recover quickly. If it turns out to be that simple, you are one of the fortunate ones. For most people it can be a long and difficult road to wellness. Be prepared for this to be a tough journey at times.

I urge you to gain some control of your own health by reading about low thyroid hormones, the various treatments, and other issues that can cause treatment to fail. I recommend that you reach out to other thyroid patients early on in your journey. This can be done via on-line patient forums and in some cases, local support groups. Many forums are on Facebook these days and others are on specialist websites like Thyroid UK, which is on a platform called HealthUnlocked. Some patients have a lot of experience. You may even find the names of excellent doctors or specialists by talking to others in your situation.

I think you should also be prepared for many work colleagues, friends and family members to not really understand what your problem actually is. This can be really disheartening and even cause friction between them and you, as they might just think that you need to 'pull yourself together'. When trying to explain to people what your condition is and how it affects you, it can be helpful to start slowly and explain what thyroid hormones actually do. Some of the coming chapters may help you to do this.

If you are in work, sadly, hypothyroidism can seriously affect your career. Trying to explain things well to your boss and Human Resources may help.

Probably the most important thing to be prepared for is the stress, frustration and setbacks that often occur when you are battling to get your condition diagnosed and treated properly. This can be soul destroying but being prepared for it should make things a little easier.

I have already said that it is important to get in the driver's seat. I believe that this is crucial for most thyroid patients if they are going to get truly well. This book is one tool to help you do that.

# Chapter 2

## Our Energy System

The next few chapters will explain how the thyroid gland and its hormones fit into an overall system. It sets the scene, so that I can talk later on about hypothyroidism and how to recover from it. I use **_our energy system_** to describe the set of glands, and entities that need to work in harmony.

When our energy system works well it allows us to move, to run, to think, to stay warm, to digest our food properly. When it works properly we are able to do everything we need to do physically and be mentally alert. Our mood is good and we interact well with others and live our lives happily.

When one part of this energy system fails, then 'all bets are off' and we begin to function poorly in many ways. If the problem is severe, it can make us bed-ridden, cold, unable to digest our food well, incapable of thinking straight or even remembering people's names. It can cause heart problems, and countless other conditions that would not otherwise have arisen. This is because our energy system affects every cell of our body and the consequences of problems can cause a vast number of symptoms.

When someone has hypothyroidism the effects can be manifold and devastating. Yet, the disease can be extremely difficult to explain to family, friends and work colleagues. Many people simply do not understand what the thyroid does. If we had diabetes or a heart problem, it would be simple to explain to a friend, colleague or family member, and have them understand and make allowances. Hypothyroidism is not as easy to describe, and people often have no clue as to how the sufferer actually feels. This is one reason why it can be so stressful and frustrating.

### What makes up our energy system?

Our energy system includes: the hypothalamus, pituitary, thyroid, adrenals, the mitochondria and the cell nuclei. They all work together to provide each cell in the body with enough thyroid hormone and energy so that all the cells can operate at the right speed and perform their unique roles.

In the coming chapters I will discuss each part of our energy system. Here is a useful analogy that may help you to understand the components of our energy system and how they relate to each other.

### The car analogy

Dr. Sarah Myhill once described something like this to me, and I have tweaked it a little.

Imagine that our body is a car. We decide what direction to go in and what speed we should be moving at. We need our car to be capable of getting us around. Sometimes we need to go faster and at other times we are happy to go at a lazy pace.

Our energy system contains critical parts in this car analogy:

- **The Hypothalamus & Pituitary glands** - the arms and legs of the driver (that control the accelerator/gas pedal & the gearbox/transmission).
- **The Thyroid gland** - the accelerator/gas pedal (requests more or less power).
- **The Adrenal glands** - the gearbox/transmission (gears-up or gears-down the engine).
- **The Mitochondria** - the engine (provides energy/power to the wheels).
- **The Cell Nuclei** - the wheels of the car (they need to 'spin' at our required rate).

Here is a simple diagram that shows the components of our energy system and some of their connections. It also refers to the **car analogy,** which I use throughout the rest of the book:

The hypothalamus controls the pituitary, and the pituitary controls both the thyroid and the adrenals (and other parts of the endocrine system beyond the scope of this book). The thyroid gland achieves its effect through thyroid hormones. Thyroid hormones stimulate the cell nuclei to perform their function faster or slower, and they also stimulate the mitochondria to produce more or less energy.

The adrenals do many things but our main interest is that they produce cortisol. The adrenals have to produce different amounts of cortisol depending on the demand, i.e. they have to be able to gear-up (or down) on demand.

Cortisol raises blood sugar levels, which the mitochondria need to produce chemical energy. The pancreas gland within our endocrine system has several functions. One of these is to make insulin. Insulin stimulates the transport of blood sugar across the cell membrane. Therefore, issues like low insulin (diabetes) and insulin resistance can wreak havoc. Cortisol also acts directly on the mitochondria to make them work faster. The mitochondria take in several important chemicals, including blood sugar, produce the much-needed fuel and deliver it to the cell nuclei. Cortisol and thyroid hormones also have powerful interactions. They need to be at appropriate levels within our cells for us to be healthy.

The cell nuclei do their particular function depending on whether they are muscle cells or brain cells or liver cells etc. The cell nuclei are like the wheels of the car - they are made to spin faster or slower based on the rest of the system.

Because the thyroid, adrenals, hypothalamus and pituitary are made of cells themselves, they also respond to thyroid hormone and cortisol.

The important thing to realise from the diagram and car analogy is that all our energy system components need to work together in harmony. The car has to be able to move at a slow or high speed when the driver requires it. If the car is not responsive, it is completely useless at getting us from one place to another in a safe and reliable way.

Having introduced the components of our energy system I will go into a little more depth on each of them, apart from the cell nuclei (which are beyond the scope of this book). I am setting the scene before talking about hypothyroidism, diagnosis and treatment. It is important to have enough background information so it is clear what happens when things go wrong and what can be done to recover.

# Chapter 3

## The Hypothalamus & Pituitary

This chapter will provide a very brief overview of the hypothalamus and pituitary glands of our energy system. In the previous chapter, I described the hypothalamus and pituitary as the arms and legs of the driver in the car analogy. They are also part of a larger system of glands known as the endocrine system.

## THE HYPOTHALAMUS

The hypothalamus is part of the brain. It is about the size of an almond and is situated below the brain stem and above the pituitary gland. Its role is to maintain internal balance in the body - known as homeostasis. The hypothalamus connects our endocrine system to our nervous system. It controls the other endocrine system glands through 'releasing' and 'inhibiting' hormones. Since the hypothalamus is connected to many parts of our brain, it is our brain that ultimately controls our hormone levels, not our hormone-producing glands, e.g. thyroid, adrenals etc.

The hypothalamus controls many important processes, including: heart rate, blood pressure, thirst, fluid and electrolyte balance, body temperature, appetite and weight gain/loss, stomach and intestinal secretions, sleep/wake cycle. The hypothalamus produces hormones that control the release of the pituitary gland's own hormones.

### Hypothalamus hormones

When our nervous system sends the hypothalamus a signal, it secretes chemicals called neuro-hormones that control the pituitary. I am not going to discuss individual hypothalamic hormones in this book. Hence, I will not list them. However, it is useful to know that many hypothalamic hormones either stimulate or inhibit the release of hormones from the pituitary gland. A few hypothalamic hormones are released directly into the posterior lobe of the pituitary, where they are released into the blood stream.

### What can go wrong with the hypothalamus's hormones?

Head injuries are known to be capable of causing problems with the hypothalamus. However, it is now thought that the more common cause of hypothalamic problems is due to brain-hypothalamic-pituitary dysfunction of unknown origin. I will often use **HP** instead of **hypothalamic-pituitary**. When I use the term **HP dysfunction** throughout this book, I mean to include *both* **HP dysfunction** (which may or may not include disease/damage to the hypothalamus or pituitary) and **HP dysregulation** (which means for some reason the HP system is not regulating one or more endocrine glands correctly, even though the hypothalamus and pituitary are both seemingly healthy glands). Hypothalamic dysfunction can result in a slight, partial or complete loss of one or more of the hypothalamic hormones. The hypothalamus controls so much of how the body works that, if it is malfunctioning, the symptoms can be so varied that it can be difficult to realise that it is the hypothalamus at fault.

If hypothalamic-pituitary (HP) dysfunction is eventually considered, most endocrinologists are usually not concerned about whether it is the hypothalamus or the pituitary gland at fault.

However, each of the pituitary hormones can be measured using blood tests. Individual, hypothalamic hormones can be given, which will detect whether the pituitary gland can respond. If the pituitary responds properly, the hypothalamus is the issue. An endocrinologist can pinpoint the source of the problem in this way, but these tests are not often carried out.

Therefore, issues in this area are frequently called hypothalamic-pituitary (HP) issues or disorders. Another common expression is hypothalamic-pituitary-adrenal axis (HPA axis), which is used when discussing the complex set of influences and feedback interactions between these three glands.

## THE PITUITARY

The pituitary gland is only about the size of a pea and is located at the base of the brain under the hypothalamus. The pituitary gland is called the 'master gland' because it controls other parts of the endocrine system: the thyroid gland, adrenals, ovaries, and testes. The hypothalamus sends hormone signals to the pituitary to stimulate or inhibit hormone production. So, the pituitary works under the control of its boss - the hypothalamus.

The pituitary is comprised of an anterior lobe (front part) and a posterior lobe (back part). The anterior lobe makes and releases hormones. The posterior lobe stores hormones that come directly from the hypothalamus and releases them into the bloodstream.

### Anterior lobe pituitary hormones

The following are stimulated by the hypothalamus:

- *Adrenocorticotropic hormone (ACTH - also called adrenocorticotropin or just corticotropin)* - ACTH stimulates the adrenal glands to produce more cortisol. ACTH also stimulates DHEA production strongly. ACTH also stimulates aldosterone, but less strongly, so reduced ACTH does not always result in aldosterone deficiency.
- *Follicle-stimulating hormone (FSH) and Luteinizing hormone (LH)* - FSH and LH work together to ensure the ovaries and testes function well, i.e. sex hormones in both cases, and the normal female monthly cycle and pregnancy. LH Stimulates the release of the highest volume of progesterone from the ovaries in the second half of a woman's cycle. LH also stimulates the production of testosterone in the testes in men and the ovaries in women.
- *Growth hormone (GH)* - GH is critical in the growth of children and in adults it is helpful in maintaining bone and muscle mass, plus it influences where fat is deposited.
- *Prolactin* - Prolactin stimulates breast milk production.

- *Thyroid-stimulating hormone (TSH)* - TSH stimulates the thyroid gland to produce hormones.

## Posterior lobe pituitary hormones

The hypothalamus releases some hormones directly into the posterior lobe. It controls this through direct connection via nerves. The pituitary then releases them. These hormones include:

- *Anti-diuretic hormone (ADH)* - ADH is used to control blood pressure and blood volume. ADH act on the kidneys and blood vessels to transport more water into the bloodstream from the kidneys. The level of ADH fluctuates to maintain blood pressure if conditions like dehydration, or even severe blood loss occur.
- *Oxytocin* - this is involved in many processes; helping us to be able to trust, to sleep, to orgasm, to control body temperature, to contract the uterus in childbirth and to produce breast milk etc.

## What can go wrong with the pituitary?

The most common cause of problems is brain-hypothalamic-pituitary dysfunction of unknown origin. Because of the difficulty of working out if the hypothalamus or pituitary are at fault I will often use the term hypothalamic-pituitary (HP) to describe these two important glands as a unit, e.g. HP dysfunction. Note: when I use the term HP-dysfunction, I implicitly mean HP-dysfunction or HP-dysregulation.

Pituitary tumours may also be a concern. They are usually benign and not life-threatening. However, they can still cause severe problems with pituitary hormone production - causing either low levels of one or more pituitary hormones or excess levels to be produced. If you had a tumour that made far too much ACTH for example, you would experience the symptoms of excess cortisol (Cushing's disease).

An accident or physical trauma can also damage the pituitary - sometimes this is temporary but it can cause permanent damage.

Clearly, the hypothalamus and pituitary are vitally important.

## Thyroid Stimulating Hormone (TSH) needs a mention now - BEWARE!

I have mentioned TSH, which is released by the pituitary to stimulate the production of thyroid hormones. When the thyroid gland produces more thyroid hormones the levels of these begin to rise in the bloodstream. The pituitary will then produce lower and less frequent pulses of TSH, causing TSH levels in the bloodstream to fall. The response of the pituitary to thyroid hormone levels is thought to be more important than the hypothalamus response, i.e. the pituitary is the gland mainly in control of the TSH level, rather than the hypothalamus.

However, TSH is not a thyroid hormone and its level has no certain connection to the actual thyroid hormone levels or to the effect of the thyroid hormone within the cells. TSH can be useful when considering the cause of hypothyroidism or hyperthyroidism. TSH on its own should *not* be used to diagnose the presence of hypothyroidism. Even a high TSH might not indicate hypothyroidism, as a person might have thyroid resistance or a TSH-secreting tumour. TSH should ***definitely not*** be used to guide treatment. As I will explain later, diagnosis and treatment should be handled using symptoms, signs and FT4 and FT3 levels - not relying on TSH very much at all.

However, over the past few decades, doctors have begun to rely on TSH for diagnosis and for dosing decisions of thyroid hormone medication - this is an utterly flawed approach. In many cases, it is the only lab test that is used to diagnose someone with hypothyroidism. Unfortunately, TSH is frequently used to check if a patient is on the right level of medication. Most doctors want to see it within the reference range (population range). This can be a huge problem for many people, as TSH is not a good indicator that someone is on the right dosage, or even the right thyroid medication!

Here are just a few problems with how TSH is often used currently:

- TSH can remain low for many years in the beginning of hypothyroidism, even though you can have many symptoms. A low TSH might convince some doctors that there were no thyroid hormone issues at all.

- Hashimoto's thyroiditis often results in fluctuating TSH that can confuse diagnosis. So, you have to be lucky when the lab test is done for the TSH to reflect your actual condition.

- Numerous research articles over recent years provide compelling evidence that TSH is not a suitable indicator of the correct dosage of thyroid hormone at all. These studies have begun to point the way to an entirely different way of assessing thyroid treatment effectiveness.

- Prior to hypothyroidism, a healthy person's thyroid hormones are produced in a rhythmic way over 24 hours. The thyroid levels fluctuate in response to TSH. This pattern of thyroid hormones over 24 hours cannot be reproduced when someone is on thyroid treatment. So, the pattern and level of your TSH is very likely to be different to when you were healthy.

- The reference ranges, used by laboratories for assessing TSH and thyroid hormone test results, are known as population ranges. They are based on the assessment of a wide population of people. However, they include the test results of thyroid patients who have been treated with thyroid medication. This makes the upper limit of the FT3 range lower than for healthy, non-thyroid patients. It also tends to make the upper limit of the FT4 range higher than for healthy, non-thyroid patients. Treated thyroid patients are often still symptomatic. They also frequently have different levels of thyroid hormones than when they were well and these affect the reference ranges. The approach of relying on assessing thyroid test results against these ranges is not sound science. More on this in Chapter 14.

- Moreover, there is good evidence to suggest that the ranges for TSH and thyroid hormones for an individual may not map neatly onto the *wide population ranges*, that are developed from assessing a population of euthyroid (apparently healthy) people. It is known from research that these *individual person references ranges* are actually much narrower (less than half as wide), and may not always fit inside the laboratory test population ranges at all. Chapter 14 discusses this further, and provides the research study reference for this.

- There is even evidence that once someone has hypothyroidism, and is on thyroid medication, that these individual person ranges may have altered from when the person was healthy, i.e. prior to developing hypothyroidism.

- There is a great deal of supporting research for all the above points and I will be referring to it later in the book. It also fits everything I have witnessed with thousands of patients over the past 10 years.

*TSH should not be used to determine whether someone is on the right type of treatment and the correct amount of it. You can be left with symptoms when TSH is relied on in this way.* This happens all too often!

There are better ways to determine if someone has hypothyroidism during treatment, through the use of symptoms, signs and actual thyroid hormone levels. Even during diagnosis, TSH should only have a supporting role. I will be discussing this extensively throughout the book.

Consequently, this is a first warning to any person who suspects that they have hypothyroidism, or if you are already undergoing treatment. Please do not fall into the mistaken idea that TSH can diagnose your problem or guide your treatment. Please do not allow your doctor to rely on this approach. It is usually not going to work and may mean that you remain sick/ill/symptomatic.

## The hypothalamus and pituitary part of our energy system

It should be obvious now why I have put this short chapter in here. The hypothalamus and pituitary are critical parts of our energy system. They are the arms and legs of the driver in the car analogy and control both the accelerator/gas pedal (the thyroid gland), and the gearbox/transmission (the adrenal glands). When things go wrong with them, we begin to have thyroid and adrenal issues. In turn, this often results in lower mitochondrial activity. This will drag our energy system down, as well as cause other serious issues.

# Chapter 4

## The Thyroid & Thyroid Hormones

The thyroid and thyroid hormones are at the centre of *The Thyroid Patient's Manual.*

The thyroid gland is located at the front of the neck just below the Adam's apple. It has two lobes and is butterfly shaped. Thyroid hormones control the metabolic rate of all our cells. The thyroid gland itself is a storage facility for thyroid hormones. The pituitary gland controls the release of these thyroid hormones via TSH.

The thyroid gland produces the hormone that is the accelerator/gas pedal within our energy system, which acts directly on the cell nuclei and mitochondria.

### THE BASICS OF HOW THE THYROID WORKS

The thyroid gland combines iodine and the amino acid tyrosine to make thyroxine (T4) and triiodothyronine (T3). T4 and T3 are then released into the blood stream and are transported to all cells throughout the body, where they control metabolism.

A protein called thyroglobulin (Tg) is produced within the thyroid. Thyroglobulin is used to hold the majority of the iodine in the thyroid. Thyroglobulin is made from the amino acid tyrosine. An enzyme called thyroid peroxidase (TPO) is also made within the thyroid. TPO is used to combine iodine and tyrosine to make all the different thyroid hormones. The thyroid hormones are stored within the thyroid gland until the TSH signal arrives from the pituitary. The TSH signal tells the thyroid to release thyroid hormones. When TSH is very low, the thyroid releases very low levels of thyroid hormones (a basal secretion). TSH stimulation is always required to lift the production and release of thyroid hormones. The thyroid gland cannot do this by itself unless it is diseased or during pregnancy.

So, we can view the thyroid gland as a factory and a warehouse for thyroid hormones. The thyroid hormones themselves are the accelerator for our energy system. The hypothalamus and pituitary can apply more pressure on the accelerator if more thyroid hormones are needed. They can ease off the accelerator if there are enough thyroid hormones or too many.

### The ratio of T4 to T3 produced by the human thyroid gland

In the American Thyroid Association's (ATA's) 2012 guidelines on the treatment of hypothyroidism, it states that approximately 85 mcg of T4 is secreted by the thyroid gland daily. Of the total daily T3 production of about 33 mcg, the majority, approximately 80% (about 26 mcg), arises from conversion from T4. Only about 20% (approximately 6.5 mcg) is produced directly by the thyroid gland.

So, if you take 85 mcg (T4 produced by the thyroid) and divide by 6.5 mcg (T3 produced by the thyroid) this gives a ratio of 13:1. This is what ATA think is produced by the thyroid; it does not take into account any conversion of T4 to T3. See **reference 10** in Resources for the research that ATA used to arrive at the 13:1 ratio.

However, thyroid researchers think that the ratio of production of T4 vs T3 is lower than 13:1, i.e. more T3 compared with the T4, but the real numbers are not known. Researchers believe that the study that ATA refer to has some issues. More research will need to be done to pin it down though. However, the ratio is **unlikely to be 4:1** as is often mentioned on the Internet and in other books.

Whatever the actual ratio is, it is by no means fixed. It is, in fact, variable and controlled. The ratio, regardless of what it is, would not help us in dosing decisions anyway.

## THE BASICS OF HOW THYROID HORMONES WORK

Thyroid hormones affect us in many ways. They are critical in the development of the foetus and growth in children. Thyroid hormones stimulate metabolic activities in most tissues of our body, which increases metabolic rate. Metabolic rate means the rate at which the cells produce and consume energy. Therefore, the thyroid gland is in charge of energy regulation in every cell of our body. This includes almost every physiological process in the body, including growth and development, metabolism, body temperature, oxygen usage and heart rate.

Thyroid hormones enter our cells via transporter proteins. Thyroid hormone can then enter the cell nuclei and bind to thyroid hormone receptors. This link up of thyroid hormone and receptor can then interact with sequences of DNA inside the nuclei. Through this mechanism, specific genes can be stimulated or turned off. This process allows thyroid hormone to affect different body tissues in different ways. For example, it can cause the heart to contract more or liver cells to perform their function faster.

Thyroid hormone also acts as a stimulant to the mitochondria, which are the engine within our energy system. I will cover the mitochondria in another chapter.

Thyroid hormones truly are the accelerator/gas pedal within our energy system, as described earlier in the car analogy. This is why, when we have a problem with the thyroid, or thyroid hormones, our entire system can be affected.

## THE THYROID HORMONES THEMSELVES

In this section, I will discuss all the hormones that the thyroid gland makes. These are: T4, T3, T2, T1 and calcitonin. I will also discuss Reverse T3 (rT3).

### Only free hormones can enter cells and be active there

The thyroid hormones T4, T3 and rT3 exist in bound and unbound forms. If bound, they are bound to protein, which renders them inactive and unable to enter cells and affect metabolism. If unbound, they are able to enter cells and affect metabolism, and are known as free hormones.

The free versions can also be written as Free-T4 (FT4) and Free-T3 (FT3). RT3 is usually assumed to be the free version when it is written that way. Blood tests for thyroid hormones are most useful when free levels are tested (total levels may be tested, but these are not very useful).

From now on when I refer to T4 and T3 and rT3, I will always mean the free levels FT4 and FT3 and rT3 - it just makes things easier to read. I only use FT4 and FT3 when I am discussing thyroid blood tests because you have to be very clear about what blood test to do.

## T4 is a pro-hormone

*T4 itself has quite a weak effect on metabolism and needs to convert to the biologically active T3 before it can be of any use.* Therefore, T4 is known as a pro-hormone or a storage hormone.

The conversion of T4 into T3 mainly occurs in the cells of the thyroid itself, the liver and kidneys. The rest is converted in the gut and in other peripheral tissues throughout the body. The T3 converted from T4 increases the level of circulating T3 in the bloodstream. Although the thyroid gland does produce some T3, most of the circulating T3 is derived from this conversion. The thyroid gland does a substantial amount of this conversion itself and it converts more than any other organ in the body.

If working correctly, there should be enough of a reservoir of the pro-hormone T4, within both the bloodstream and the cells, for future conversion to T3. However, many problems can prevent T4 from converting to enough T3.

## T3 is the biologically active thyroid hormone

T4 converts to both T3 and rT3, in about equal proportions, in a healthy person.

T3 binds more readily to the nuclear thyroid receptors than T4. Researchers have found that T3 is 10-15 times more likely to bind with the thyroid receptors than T4. *Moreover, the action of T3 within the cell nuclei is 10 times more powerful than that of T4.* T4 does bind to thyroid receptors at the cell membrane, where it exerts some effects. However, these are still far less significant than the T3 effects at the cell nuclei.

*It is essential to understand that it is the T3 thyroid hormone that is most biologically active within our cells.* Moreover, T3 can only be useful once it is *inside the cells.* It does nothing at all in the bloodstream.

So, when I discuss the *effect of thyroid hormone(s)* from now on, I implicitly mean that it is the *T3 thyroid hormone* that is causing this effect - not the pro-hormone T4. Remember, only T3 has any substantial biological effect in the body. T4 itself is barely a hormone at all.

Note: medical science cannot measure how much actual T3 gets inside each type of cell in the body (it has been done in rat studies but requires dissection to do it). Therefore, doctors can only assess blood levels and these frequently do not reflect actual metabolic activity. The only way to assess how T3 is affecting metabolism, is to observe how someone has responded to treatment in terms of their *symptoms* and other things like body temperature, heart rate, weight change (these measurable parameters are sometimes called *signs*). When a doctor assesses the symptoms and signs of a patient, and how these are changing through thyroid treatment, they are assessing the *clinical* situation.

## Reverse T3

T4 converts to a mixture of T3 and rT3. This process of conversion to rT3 occurs on an on-going basis within the cells, in order to clear excess levels of T4 from the body, or to lower metabolic rate in certain circumstances. RT3 is eventually broken down and converted into T2, which in turn is converted into T1. The body then eliminates T1 within 24 hours.

RT3 acts like a metabolic brake in the cell nuclei and can slow down metabolism - the opposite of FT3. However, this effect is not noticeable unless there is too much rT3 present. In this latter situation, the person can feel hypothyroid. There is research that clearly shows that rT3 is a brake on the effect of T3 (see *reference 4* listed in Resources at the end of the chapter). However, many doctors still hold the view that rT3 does nothing at all, and is simply an inactive metabolite. This is just plain wrong. Unfortunately, this belief is largely why many doctors do not wish to test rT3 at all.

RT3 exists to provide a means to match the available T3 to the body's actual needs. Some studies show that most people convert over 50% of their T4 to rT3. So, they convert less than 50% of T4 to the metabolically active T3. The levels of rT3 fluctuate up and down throughout the day. Therefore, it is impossible to specify an ideal level for rT3 or any ideal ratio of FT3 to rT3. However, we do know that low FT3 and high rT3 is likely to slow metabolism.

RT3 also provides a mechanism for slowing down the metabolism in the event of starvation, serious illness or high stress. In these circumstances the conversion rate of T4 to T3 decreases and more rT3 is made. The reduced T3 level that occurs during illness, fasting, or stress slows the metabolism of most of the cells of the body.

## T2 and T1 thyroid hormones

I have explained that T3 is produced through the deiodination of T4. T3 is also subject to deiodination within the cells. It is through the deiodination of T3, that more T2 and T1 are produced. T2 and T1 are also present in the thyroid gland, and are released into the bloodstream. However, the vast majority of T2 and T1 is produced directly from T3. Research is still discovering the exact functions of both of these hormones.

If someone is taking T3 medication, they will get adequate amounts of T2 and T1.

## Calcitonin

Calcitonin is also produced by the thyroid gland. It is involved in helping to regulate the levels of calcium and phosphate in the body. It opposes the action of the parathyroid glands, which control the body's calcium level. The Society of Endocrinologists have concluded that there is little effect on the body of either moderately high calcitonin or too little. Patients who have had their thyroid gland removed have no calcitonin in their blood and show no adverse symptoms as a result.

## METABOLISM AND ACTION OF THYROID HORMONES

### T4 to T3 conversion

T4 to T3 conversion occurs within every cell of the body. Most of the T3 in the blood comes from conversion within the cells of the thyroid gland, liver, kidneys, peripheral tissues and the gastrointestinal tract.

All cells depend on taking some T3 from the bloodstream and/or taking in T4 and converting it to T3. The cells vary substantially in their ability to convert T4 to T3 depending on what tissue they are part of.

This process of conversion requires the removal of an iodine atom from a T4 molecule, so it is referred to as deiodination. There are enzymes produced in certain tissues (cells of the body), called deiodinase enzymes. It is through the action of two of these enzymes (D1 and D2 deiodinase) that T4 is converted to T3. The brain, pituitary, heart, thyroid and skeleton muscle (peripheral tissues) use D2 to convert T4 to T3. The liver, kidneys and thyroid use D1. D2 is significantly more efficient in converting T4 to T3 than D1. However, D1 deiodinase is very important in the clearance of rT3 by the liver. The liver clears rT3 through deiodination of rT3 into T2, then T1 and T0 (which is excreted within a day). In some people, genetic defects associated with these enzymes can hamper conversion from T4 to T3 and rT3 clearance.

*The thyroid gland contributes 25% of our circulating T3.* This occurs through T3 production and T4 to T3 conversion within the thyroid. Consequently, the thyroid production of T3, and its conversion of T4 to T3, provides a large proportion of the available T3 in the body. Even if the thyroid gland produced no hormones of its own, it would still convert the T4 that is present in the blood that flows through it. *The thyroid gland is like a little machine that sits in the blood flow, converting T4 to T3.* Hence, achieving good symptom relief with T4-Only therapy after both thyroidectomy and long-term Hashimoto's is often very difficult. This explains why so many of these people require additional T3 alongside T4. Research studies back all of this up. *After total thyroidectomy, patients lose around 25% of their total circulating T3.* See *references 11, 12* in Resources.

The gastrointestinal tract is also responsible for some of the conversion of T4 to T3, but it only happens if the gut is healthy and has the right level of friendly gut bacteria.

T4 to T3 conversion requires adequate amounts of the right deiodinase enzymes and these are heavily dependent on the mineral selenium in their construction. Consequently, it is important to have enough selenium in the diet or through supplements. The conversion process is also dependent on levels of zinc, ferritin, selenium and iodine.

The activity of the D1 and D2 deiodinase enzymes involved in conversion does not occur at a fixed rate; it is variable, but regulated. There are a variety of studies that prove that the *level of TSH that is present in the bloodstream affects the conversion rate of T4 to T3.* This is certainly true within the thyroid and the liver - which do most of the conversion. *A higher level of TSH will increase the conversion rate of T4 to T3. A lower level of TSH will reduce the conversion rate*. These points can be important when it comes to managing thyroid hormone replacement. I will discuss this further in Chapter 7. This is a crucial point though. Conversion from T4 to T3 does not just happen at a fixed rate; TSH regulates it. There are several studies that show this - see *references 5,6,7 and 8* in Resources.

### T3 has to reach its targets for us to feel healthy

It is absolutely essential that enough T3 reach the cell nuclei and the mitochondria. If this does not happen, our metabolism will suffer and we will not remain healthy.

The T3 thyroid hormone binds to receptors in both the mitochondria and the cell nuclei.

T3 acts on the mitochondria to stimulate more energy production.

The action of T3 thyroid hormone on the genes within the cell nuclei is the most significant way in which thyroid hormone affects the tissues. This is known as the genomic action of T3. Thousands of genes within the cell nuclei can be turned on or off. The response of the genes to T3 may take hours, days, weeks or longer to fully occur. Because of the length of time it can take to restructure the genes, it is important to be patient when someone is trying to recover from hypothyroidism. Sometimes, treatment cannot be rushed quickly because of this.

## WHAT CAN GO WRONG WITH THE THYROID SYSTEM

Lots can go wrong with the thyroid gland and with the hormones themselves. Even more can go wrong when we look at other factors that can affect our energy system. A good portion of this book will be devoted to outlining these things, how to test for them and how to deal with them. Here, I am strictly concentrating on the thyroid gland and its hormones.

The focus of this book is hypothyroidism. Hypothyroidism has been classically, but incorrectly defined, as insufficient T4 and T3 thyroid hormones. It is also sometimes called Underactive Thyroid or simply Low Thyroid. However, if the action of the thyroid hormone T3 is inadequate to regulate metabolism, this is still hypothyroidism (this broadens the definition to include syndromes like thyroid hormone resistance). I will therefore use an improved and far clearer definition of hypothyroidism.

### My use of the term hypothyroidism

From this chapter, it should be clear that the cause of hypothyroid symptoms is due to the sub-optimal effect of the biologically active T3 within some or all of the cells.

Many things can cause this. Some examples are:

- Low cortisol, or more properly, hypocortisolism, as cortisol and T3 work together.
- Total thyroidectomy or Hashimoto's thyroiditis (causing thyroid gland damage) - both result in too little T3 (including the T3 converted from T4 by the thyroid gland).
- Poor conversion of T4 to T3.
- Some form of thyroid hormone resistance.
- Central hypothyroidism, resulting in insufficient TSH, and therefore, low T4 and T3.

However, it is the sub-optimal effect of T3 within some or all of the tissues that causes the symptoms associated with hypothyroidism (for whatever reason there is not enough T3-effect).

So, when I use the term *hypothyroidism* from now on I mean *the sub-optimal effect of T3 thyroid hormone within some or all of the cells of the body*. It includes everything that stops T3 from optimally operating within the cells. Some of the issues that result in hypothyroidism may not be visible on any current medical test. It is a more precise definition and is far less ambiguous than low thyroid hormone.

### Further classification of hypothyroidism

Where hypothyroidism is caused by the failure of a gland, it can be classified further:

- *Primary hypothyroidism* - where the thyroid gland fails to produce enough T4 and T3. This is the most common type of hypothyroidism.
- *Secondary hypothyroidism* - is less common and occurs if the pituitary gland itself fails to produce enough TSH.
- *Tertiary hypothyroidism* - is due to a fault within the hypothalamus gland.
- *Central hypothyroidism* - is a collective term for both secondary and tertiary hypothyroidism.

### Symptoms of hypothyroidism include:

| | |
|---|---|
| Fatigue/tiredness/needing more sleep | Feeling cold/cold hands or feet |
| Low body temperature | Myxoedema (swollen skin) |
| Weak muscles/muscle cramps | Weight gain |
| Slow movement | Constipation |
| Depression | Thin, brittle, cracked fingernails |
| Coarse hair/hair loss/outer eyebrow loss | Dry, coarse, itchy skin, acne, skin infections |
| Decreased libido | Irritability, mood swings |
| Low heart rate/heart palpitations | Poor memory |
| Impaired thinking ability (brain fog) | Lack of concentration |
| Headaches or migraines | Joint pain or muscle pain or fibromyalgia |
| Swallowing problems/swollen tongue | Loss of appetite |
| Changes in voice (slower, rougher) | Tinnitus |
| Abnormal or painful menstrual cycles | Anaemia |
| Water retention | Sluggish reflexes |
| Shortness of breath, laboured breathing | Insomnia |
| Allergies | Cold intolerance/heat intolerance |
| High blood pressure | Sometimes low blood pressure |
| Tension/anxiety | Heart problems |
| Hypoglycaemia (low blood sugar) | Vertigo |

If extreme iodine deficiency is a cause of the hypothyroidism, the thyroid can become very large and it is called a goitre. This problem used to be less common, as iodine supplementation of salt reduced its frequency. However, many people are now using sea salt, which usually does not have added iodine. So the problem may be becoming more common again.

## Hashimoto's Thyroiditis

Hashimoto's is an autoimmune disorder that over time will destroy the entire thyroid gland. As it progresses, hypothyroid symptoms will begin to present themselves as the level of thyroid hormones begins to fall. Sometimes symptoms may oscillate between hypothyroid and hyperthyroid symptoms (because far too much thyroid hormone may get released into the bloodstream as the thyroid tissue gets destroyed). The latter condition makes treatment a lot more complex.

## Hashimoto's thyroiditis autoantibodies

When Hashimoto's thyroiditis is present, one or more of the following autoantibodies will be present:

- *Thyroid peroxidase antibody (TPOAb)* - this is the most common autoantibody to be raised in Hashimoto's - with about 90% of Hashi's patients showing raised levels. The TPOAb autoantibodies are markers that indicate that the immune system is causing damage to the thyroid cells, and high levels of TPOAb often precede thyroid gland destruction (which can take many years to occur).

- *Thyroglobulin antibody (TgAb)* - these autoantibodies are often raised in Hashimoto's thyroiditis - with around 80% of Hashi's patients having raised levels. This autoantibody is unnecessary to test if TPOAb is already positive.

- *Thyroid stimulating hormone receptor antibody (TRAb)* - this refers to the receptors in the thyroid gland that respond to the stimulus of TSH from the pituitary gland. These autoantibodies may be raised in Hashimoto's thyroiditis. TRAb is often raised in Graves' disease; another type of autoimmune thyroid disorder that causes high levels of thyroid hormones to be produced.

- I spoke to one thyroid patient who had *TSH-Receptor Blocking Antibodies (TRBAb)*, which blocked TSH from reaching the thyroid receptors. She described it to me as a reverse Graves's disease, which causes hypothyroidism and thyroid gland atrophy over time, due to lack of TSH stimulation. This is not Hashimoto's; it is more rare, but is still worth mentioning. See *reference 13* in Resources.

Usually your family doctor will determine which of the autoantibodies to test for and how frequently to do the tests, based on your medical history.

However, I urge anyone with suspected hypothyroidism to request that their doctor tests TPOAb at the outset, as this is the most common autoantibody to be raised. If TPOAb is negative, TgAb should be tested. If one of these were raised, you would have an opportunity to attempt to halt Hashimoto's thyroiditis. I have listed Izabella Wentz's excellent book on this subject in the Resources at the end of the chapter. Even if you were not able to halt its progress, at least you would be prepared for further thyroid deterioration (and the likely need for further increases in thyroid medication over time). Note: the use of chelated selenium (100-200 mg per day) is thought to be of benefit to halting Hashimoto's thyroiditis and in helping generally with thyroid function and conversion of T4 to T3.

## Reduced T4 to T3 Conversion

If for any reason the conversion rate of T4 to T3 is reduced, you will have a lower FT3 level than when you were healthy and fit. This means that the biologically active thyroid hormone is present in less volume in the blood and in the cells. If your doctor tests FT3 and the result falls within the reference range, your doctor might mistakenly assume that everything is fine. It is important to know that even though your FT3 level may fall within the reference range, you will probably not know your FT3 level when you were well. It could have fallen from a much higher level. Being in the reference range for FT3 does not stop someone from having thyroid symptoms. This is one of the huge problems in the current handling of hypothyroidism.

If your conversion rate of T4 to T3 has reduced, the T4 is often converted to rT3 instead. Lower FT3 and higher rT3, combine to make the metabolism far slower.

There are many causes of reduced T4 to T3 conversion. Here are just a few:

- *Genetic defects* - in May 2009 a group of researchers (Panicker, V. et al) in the UK published the WATTS Study (Western Area T4/T3 Study - it was done in the west of England, and involved one of my ex-endos, now Professor Colin Dayan). See *reference 9* in the Resources for the link to this study. This is the largest and most comprehensive study to date, of hypothyroid patients treated with combination T4 and T3. The researchers looked at 697 hypothyroid individuals and analysed their DNA for differences in the deiodinase enzymes. The study found that there is a substantial difference among individuals in the genes that make the deiodinases. Genetic mutations can make some people far less effective in converting T4 to T3. They found that around 16% of people in the study had two copies of the faulty DIO2 deiodinase gene, which means they could not make a normal D2 enzyme. This would suggest that some people would never do well on conventional thyroid treatment with just T4 medication. Also since the conversion occurs within cells and not all of the T3 will be returned to the bloodstream, *poor conversion may never show up on any thyroid blood test panel*. Note: *Regenerus Labs.* can test for this DIO2 faulty gene (which is the most important one). You can also look for the *DIO1 and DIO2 mutations* in the raw data from genome analysis companies. However, please check they do test for these mutations first before buying the test kit. Some do and some do not. I have had *DIO2* tested myself, and I am positive for the homozygous variant of the DIO2 gene, having inherited from both my mother and father, i.e. I have two copies.

I also have two copies of the *DIO1* defect. Mutations of the deiodinase enzymes that reduce their function are common - not rare! The DIO mutations discovered so far may be the tip of the iceberg of deiodinase dysfunction. This may be one of the arguments you can use to persuade your doctor to add T3 to your treatment, if T4 treatment is not working well.

- *Cortisol (high and low) - high cortisol* levels reduce TSH secretion and T4 to T3 conversion. This is something that I have seen many times through correspondence with thyroid patients. It frequently catapults them into hypothyroidism due to induced low FT3 levels, and higher rT3 levels. Prolonged stress, of course, can be a cause of this and the commencement of hypothyroidism. Usually, this period of high cortisol does not last long and it eventually turns into low cortisol. *Low cortisol* can also impact conversion, as this will have a direct effect on mitochondrial activity, which will become apparent over the next two chapters. Low cortisol also impacts T3-effect in the cells and reduces the ability for T3 to bind to the thyroid receptors. Low cortisol is far more common than high cortisol and it will be discussed many times within this book. I also had extremely low cortisol. Low cortisol often responds to adding T3 to treatment. So, again this might be something you can discuss with your doctor when trying to get some T3 added to your treatment.

- *Loss of thyroid tissue* - through thyroidectomy or long-term Hashimoto's. The thyroid gland converts more T4 to T3 than any other tissue in the body. In the early stages of Hashimoto's, TSH will rise because thyroid tissue is being destroyed. This will mask the disease for a while, as the higher TSH will increase the conversion rate of T4 to T3. However, over time, the loss of thyroid tissue will result in the loss of a significant amount of the T4 to T3 conversion that occurs on the T4 carried by the blood flowing through the gland. If you have lost a lot of thyroid tissue through a thyroidectomy or Hashimoto's, adding some T3 to your treatment may be necessary to compensate for this loss of conversion. Remember, your thyroid accounts for 25% of your total circulating T3, including conversion capability. The thyroid converts more T4 than any other organ.

- *Sex hormones* - low or imbalanced sex hormones that often occur during peri-menopause and menopause may cause cortisol issues, through HP-dysfunction. If the sex hormone issue is not detected, any cortisol problem may be difficult to resolve and continue to contribute to conversion issues from T4 to T3. I will discuss this further in Chapter 21.

- *Epigenetic changes* - this crudely means that genes can be switched on or off through prolonged changes in the biological status of an individual. Some of these genetic changes can be very hard to reverse. Consider the case of someone who has had undiagnosed hypothyroidism for some time. If a doctor eventually decides to treat this patient with T4, there may now be a conversion issue. Having been hypothyroid for a long time, the patient is now in a different state, compared to the previous healthy state. Epigenetic changes are well documented. Regaining health can be a long drawn out process, because epigenetic changes through illness are not quickly reversed. So, simply having free thyroid hormones, or TSH, sitting within a reference range is no guarantee of being correctly treated. Even if all the right conditions can be met to reverse the changes, it can take six months or longer to change back, because the new person has to be built from scratch, so to speak.

- *Low levels of nutrients* - it is known that low levels of important nutrients, e.g. selenium, iron etc., can also contribute to a reduced T4 to T3 conversion rate.

## All current medicine can do is to test what is in the blood

The levels of FT4, and especially FT3, in the bloodstream do not always reflect the levels within the cells where the hormones are active. My first book *Recovering with T3* spends much of its time on this topic. It is one of the crucial things of which all thyroid patients should be aware.

There are many things that can go wrong within the actual cells. Much of this is beyond the capability of current medicine to test or reveal. Since T4 to T3 conversion occurs within the cells of the body, there can be a deficiency of T3 there. This intracellular T3 level cannot be tested. Intracellular resistance to T3 can also cause poor-effect of T3 within the cells, which is undetectable by a test. However, doctors often deem any FT3 blood test result (low or otherwise) that is inside the reference range to be normal! Many doctors do not even think testing FT3 (the active thyroid hormone) is required at all. Very few doctors are willing to prescribe T3 to correct hypothyroidism (which I have already defined as sub-optimal effect of T3 within the cells - which your doctor cannot test for).

The reference range for each thyroid lab test result is a range that applies to a large population. However, many laboratories include the data from thyroid patients with in-range TSH levels to construct the reference ranges. These patients are not screened out for symptoms and should not be included in the construction of the reference ranges used for diagnosis and treatment. *This inevitably lowers the top of the reference range for FT3* (and tends to raise the top of the reference range for FT4). If only healthy non-thyroid patients were used to construct the reference ranges, they would not be as skewed.

It is also known from recent research that each individual person has a unique normal or *person range* for each thyroid hormone. These unique person ranges are thought to be less than half as wide as the population/reference range, and may not map neatly onto the reference/ range. This is a big issue, which I will return to, and provide research evidence for.

Conventional medical practices for the replacement of thyroid hormones can result in thyroid levels that appear normal on blood tests. Many doctors conclude that persistent hypothyroid symptoms are not related to the hormone therapy because of this. Patients are frequently left with symptoms, and are often told that they have some other issue. This is so sad, because it is so avoidable.

## RESOURCES

Here is a list of further reading for those who wish to gather more background on the thyroid, thyroid hormones and Hashimoto's:

1. *Solved The Riddle of Illness* - Stephen Langer, M.D., and James F. Scheer.

2. *Hypothyroidism Type 2* - Mark Starr, M.D. (probably my favourite book as an introduction to hypothyroidism).

3. *Hashimoto's Thyroiditis* - Izabella Wentz, PharmD, FASCP.

4. *Qualitative and quantitative differences in the pathways of extrathyroidal triiodothyronine generation between euthyroid and hypothyroid rats* - J E Silva, M B Gordon, F R Crantz, J L Leonard, and P R Larsen.
   See: https://www.jci.org/articles/view/111313 (This paper shows that rT3 is a T3 blocker and is not an inactive metabolite).

5. *Relational stability in the expression of normality, variation, and control of thyroid function* - Hoermann R, Midgley JEM, Larisch R, Dietrich JW. See: Front Endocrinol (2016) 7:57–8. doi:10.3389/fendo.2016.00142

6. *Regulation of Thyroidal Deiodinase Activity* - Conti, A., Studer, H., Kneubuehl, F., Kohler, See: H. Endocrinology, Vol. 102 (1):321-329, 1978.

7. *Effect of thyrotropin on conversion of T4 to T3 in perfused rat liver* - Ikeda, K., Takeuchi, T., Ito, Y., Murakami, I., Mokuda, O., Tominaga, M., Mashiba, H. See: Life Sciences, Volume 38, Issue 20:1801-1806, 1986

8. *Effect of TSH on conversion of T4 to T3 in perfused rat kidney* - Ikeda, T., Honda M., Murakami, I., Kuno, S., Mokuda, O., Tokumori, Y., Tominaga, M., Mashiba, H. See: Metabolism, Volume 34, Issue 11:1057-1060, 1985.

9. *Common variation in the DIO2 gene predicts baseline psychological well-being and response to combination T4/T3 therapy in patients on thyroid hormone replacement* - Vijay Panicker, Ponnusamy Saravanan, Bijay Vaidya, Jonathan Evans, Andrew T. Hattersley, Timothy M. Frayling and Colin M. Dayan. See: The Journal of Clinical Endocrinology & Metabolism Vol. 94, No. 5 1623-1629 (2009)

10. *The AACE/ATA guidelines quote a complicated study by Pilo in 1990 for their claim of 13:1 T4:T3 thyroid hormone production* -
    See: https://www.ncbi.nlm.nih.gov/pubmed/2333963

11. *Dual control of pituitary thyroid stimulating hormone secretion by thyroxine and triiodothyronine in athyreotic patients* - Hoermann R, Midgley JEM, Dietrich JW, Larisch R.
    Seee: The Adv Endocrinol Metab (2017) 8:83–95. doi:10.1177/2042018817716401

12. *Relational stability of thyroid hormones in euthyroid subjects and patients with autoimmune thyroid disease* - Hoermann R, Midgley JEM, Larisch R, Dietrich JW.
    See: Eur Thyroid J (2016) 5:171–179. doi:10.1159/000447967

13. *Atrophic Thyroiditis* - by Luis J. Jara, which is a section in the book Diagnostic Criteria in Autoimmune Diseases.
    See: https://link.springer.com/chapter/10.1007%2F978-1-60327-285-8_42

# Chapter 5

## The Adrenals & Adrenal Hormones

The two adrenal glands, each the size of a walnut, sit on top of the kidneys. The hormones that they produce are critical for life. The adrenals have both a cortex (outer part) that makes several hormones and a medulla (central part).

The adrenal medulla of each adrenal gland produces adrenaline, which is the hormone that is produced in the 'fight or flight' response. It is the hormone that enables you to immediately cope with stress, anger and fear.

The adrenal cortex of each adrenal gland makes many of its steroid hormones from cholesterol. It converts cholesterol into pregnenolone, which it then converts into other steroid hormones. See *reference 4* in Resources at the end of the chapter, for a clear and comprehensive diagram that shows the biochemical pathways involved in making steroid hormones in the adrenal cortices, the gonads (ovaries and testes) and in other tissues.

The main hormones produced in the adrenal cortices are:
- Cortisol.
- Aldosterone.
- The weak androgens - DHEA and androstenedione.
- Pregnenolone.
- Some progesterone.
- Testosterone - but only a small amount.

DHEA and its inactive sulfate, DHEAS, are the most abundant steroids in the body. DHEA can be converted within tissues into androgens and oestrogens, and eventually into testosterone and oestradiol.

DHEA is critical to our health, as it counteracts and balances cortisol's effects throughout the body. DHEA and androstenedione help the body to repair itself. In women who still have monthly cycles, about 50% of the testosterone in the bloodstream is derived from adrenal DHEA. DHEAS can be converted to DHEA, so it is also important.

Aldosterone signals the kidneys to retain salt and water, thus maintaining the body's fluid and electrolyte (sodium and potassium) balance. Aldosterone is therefore critical to regulating blood pressure.

*ACTH from the pituitary gland stimulates the secretion of all these steroids (cortisol, DHEA, androstenedione and to a lesser extent aldosterone).*

Aldosterone secretion is also stimulated by the renin-angiotensin system in the kidneys. The renin-angiotensin system is a hormone system that regulates blood pressure and fluid balance. Therefore, insufficient ACTH production causes both cortisol and DHEAS to be low, but does not usually result in a significant aldosterone deficiency.

Note: it is worth mentioning that the adrenal glands and the way that they work is much the same for both women and men.

I will discuss more about the adrenal glands and their relationship with sex hormones in Chapter 21.

However, the main hormone that I want to discuss is cortisol, which is produced in high volume by the adrenal glands.

## THE BASICS OF WHAT CORTISOL DOES

Cortisol has several functions in the body. It raises the level of blood sugar by causing the release of glucose that has been stored in various other forms in the body. High levels of cortisol can also raise blood pressure, and low levels can reduce blood pressure. More cortisol is produced in times of intense stress, in order to protect us from any adverse effects.

Cortisol has a suppressive effect on the immune system and prevents the release of substances that cause inflammation. So, cortisol restrains the immune system. Low cortisol promotes allergies and autoimmune disease. Cortisol also has a role in the processing of fat, protein and carbohydrate within the body.

Cortisol may be viewed as having the opposite effect to insulin. Insulin's role is to make our cells more receptive to the glucose that they need and to help store any excess blood glucose within the liver, muscles and fat tissues. Cortisol tends to keep glucose at a good level in the bloodstream.

Cortisol is important to the mitochondria for two reasons. Firstly, it ensures there is enough blood glucose, which the mitochondria require so that they can perform their role. Secondly, cortisol is a direct stimulant of mitochondrial activity.

Keep in mind that even if cortisol enables a good level of glucose in the bloodstream, this will not get into the cells unless there is enough insulin and there is no insulin resistance.

Cortisol enhances the effect of biologically active T3 thyroid hormone within our cells. T3 and cortisol have powerful interactions and both need to be at good levels for us to be healthy.

So, cortisol is our stress-coping hormone. Sufficient cortisol levels/effects are vital to a person's quality of life and ability to function under stress. Without sufficient cortisol-effects we suffer from fatigue, poor recovery from stress or exertion, cognitive dysfunction, pain, anxiety, depression, allergies and autoimmune disease.

Even if there is no ACTH secretion, the adrenals will continue to produce a low level of cortisol

It should be clear that the adrenals have to 'gear-up' to support the changing needs for cortisol. Hence, in the car analogy, the adrenals are the gearbox/transmission within our energy system (probably the weakest part of this analogy but no analogy is perfect!). Importantly, if you are in the wrong gear, the accelerator/gas pedal does not have the desired effect.

## Cortisol production over 24-hours

The adrenal glands produce cortisol throughout the day and night. The largest amount of cortisol is produced in the last 4 hours of sleep, typically between the hours of 4:00 a.m. and 8:00 a.m., depending on the individual's sleep/wake cycle. It reaches its peak usually when we first wake up. Then, during the day, less and less cortisol is produced and levels slowly reduce. Cortisol is normally at its lowest level in the evening when we are getting ready to sleep. It may drop to around 10% of the morning peak level.

This is the normal daily pattern of cortisol, which can be referred to as its circadian rhythm. If someone has a very different pattern of sleeping and being awake, or there are other problems, the timing of cortisol release will be different. Different timings of cortisol can cause big issues for the individual.

If during the day we are involved in any increased stress or big physical activity, our energy system works together to request more cortisol.

Cortisol production is also affected by the quality of sleep that we get. Deep sleep produces a normal, optimal morning cortisol rise.

## ADDISON'S DISEASE

Addison's disease is a life-threatening condition. ***Proceeding with thyroid treatment without diagnosing and treating Addison's disease could risk an Addisonian crisis and death.*** So, I am going to deal with Addison's disease now, and after that concern myself with the less serious and more common issues that thyroid patients often have.

In ***Addison's disease*** the adrenal cortices are destroyed. This is usually caused by autoimmune attack. In this case, ACTH is not effective in producing sufficient cortisol.

***Sufficient cortisol*** is required to maintain health and quality of life. In states of physiological stress, particularly caused by infection or physical exertion, the body produces significantly more cortisol - sometimes even by a factor of 10. Consequently, in Addison's disease the body cannot meet the demand for higher cortisol, and an Addisonian crisis can result, which can be life-threatening.

***Sufficient aldosterone*** is required to maintain blood pressure and sodium/potassium balance. Many deaths from Addisonian crisis, or adrenal crisis, are caused by nearly complete absence of aldosterone, which is necessary to maintain blood pressure and sodium/potassium levels and balance. Potassium levels become very high and can cause cardiac arrhythmias.

Note: in central adrenal insufficiency (little or no ACTH stimulation), the cortices will continue to produce sufficient aldosterone in most individuals. They will also produce a little cortisol - even with no ACTH secretion at all.

Addison's disease is extremely serious and must be ruled out **before** proceeding with thyroid treatment if there is any evidence for it being present. To begin thyroid treatment in the presence of undiagnosed Addison's would risk causing an Addisonian crisis.

**Addison's disease symptoms usually develop slowly over many months:**

| | |
|---|---|
| Extreme fatigue | Weight loss and decreased appetite |
| Darkening of your skin (hyperpigmentation) | Low blood pressure, fainting, worse on standing |
| Salt craving | Low blood sugar (hypoglycaemia) |
| Nausea, diarrhoea or vomiting | Abdominal pain |
| Muscle or joint pains | Irritability |
| Low mood, mild depression | Body hair loss or sexual dysfunction on women |
| Frequent urination | Drowsiness |
| Increased thirst | Dehydration |

If some or all of these symptoms are not responded to, the situation can worsen over time. These symptoms typically worsen when even a mild illness like a cold occurs.

Eventually, either because of the situation not being dealt with, or through more physiological stress (typically physical exertion or infection), an Addisonian crisis can occur.

**Acute adrenal failure/Addisonian crisis symptoms:**

| | |
|---|---|
| Pain in your lower back, abdomen or legs | Severe vomiting/diarrhoea |
| Low blood pressure, worse when standing up | Severe drowsiness or loss of consciousness |
| High potassium and low sodium | Muscle cramps |
| Severe dehydration | Pale, cold and clammy skin |
| Sweating | Rapid, shallow breathing |
| Severe muscle weakness | Headache |

If the above is not promptly attended to, the risk of death through an Addisonian crisis is significantly higher.

## Addison's disease needs to be diagnosed and treated by an endocrinologist

This needs to be diagnosed and treated by an endocrinologist, as it can be life-threatening as I have said many times now. Extremely low cortisol in Addison's disease, is treated with hydrocortisone (HC), which is bio-identical cortisol.

Once on HC treatment, the individual needs to be aware that there are situations where a higher HC dosage needs to be used. The reason for this is that the HC an Addison's patient requires will fully suppress any remaining ability to make cortisol. So, in the event of higher physiological stress, the body cannot respond to it by making more cortisol. The need has to be met by using more HC medication. The endocrinologist should have fully briefed the Addison's patient that they need to carry emergency stress doses of HC with them. Being fully aware of all the potential issues and how to deal with them is essential for an Addison's patient.

*It is not a disease to be treated without expert help.*

*If your doctor suspects severe hypocortisolism, or adrenal gland damage or low aldosterone you need to be referred to an endocrinologist for further investigation.*

Severe hypocortisolism may also prompt the doctor to consider low aldosterone as a possible problem, as this is often also present in Addison's disease.

*Low aldosterone* is often suggested by low blood pressure, lower blood pressure on standing, low sodium and high potassium or low aldosterone symptoms. Aldosterone and renin tests are often run to confirm this. Sometimes a trial of fludrocortisone (Florinef) is given to see how the individual responds.

If Addison's disease is diagnosed, cortisol and aldosterone must be replaced first and brought to a healthy level. This needs to happen *before any thyroid hormone replacement.* Otherwise, starting thyroid hormone replacement can trigger an Addisonian crisis.

*This book will not be covering the diagnosis or treatment protocol for Addison's disease or for dealing with low aldosterone.*

I have included a link to an Addison's support group - see *reference 1* in Resources at the end of the chapter. I have also included some guidance on what to do if someone is already on HC and they need to respond to adrenal emergencies - see *reference 5* in Resources.

## WHAT ELSE CAN GO WRONG WITH THE ADRENAL SYSTEM

The rest of this chapter assumes that your doctor or endocrinologist has *excluded Addison's disease, with the severely low cortisol and low aldosterone.*

Many thyroid patients experience the milder levels of low cortisol, sometimes known as partial adrenal insufficiency, or adrenal fatigue. Both of these terms are misleading, as I will discuss soon.

Some of the symptoms of hypothyroidism may be confused with some of the symptoms of low cortisol, since both can lower metabolic rate. As previously mentioned, low cortisol may interfere with the conversion of T4 to T3, and result in lower FT3 and elevated rT3. Low cortisol also reduces T3-effect in the cells. When cortisol is low, blood sugar may also be low. Insufficient blood sugar will slow down the mitochondria - thus slowing down the metabolism.

If someone has been experiencing high levels of emotional or physical stress for a long time, their adrenal glands may begin to produce less cortisol. This may also be true for the person who has been hypothyroid for several years before diagnosis and treatment. Low cortisol may also result from exposure to environmental toxins, dietary sensitivities and allergens, as well as traumatic life events.

## Hypothalamic-pituitary (HP) dysfunction

The mechanism that most frequently causes low cortisol is hypothalamic-pituitary (HP) dysfunction. In Chapter 3, I made it clear that when I used the term *HP dysfunction* I also mean to include *HP dysregulation* (which means that for some reason the HP system is not controlling one or more endocrine glands correctly, even though there may be no damage or disease in either the hypothalamus or pituitary). I will not define this again.

Contrary to what many alternative medicine practitioners claim, the adrenal glands do not become 'fatigued' or 'tired'. They can continue to make and secrete cortisol in large amounts as long as they are stimulated to do so by sufficient ACTH from the pituitary gland. For instance, cortisol levels remain very high indefinitely in Cushing's disease - when a tumour produces excessive ACTH. So, even in the state of constant and prolonged excessive cortisol production, the adrenals just keep making cortisol. The adrenals can continue to make all the steroid hormones as long as there is sufficient cholesterol in the blood. The rate-limiting step in cortisol production is the amount of ACTH-stimulation of the adrenal cortices. Hence, the terms 'adrenal fatigue' or 'tired adrenals' are misleading. The term 'partial adrenal insufficiency' tends to imply that the adrenals are 'partially insufficient'. It is a vague term, but it is misleading too, as the adrenals themselves are usually not the issue. We need a more precise description.

It is also worth knowing that we cannot increase cortisol levels by supplying precursors in the blood, e.g. by taking pregnenolone or progesterone. Even in the presence of low cholesterol, these precursors make no difference in cortisol levels. Cortisol is rate-limited by ACTH. See *reference 6* in Resources at the end of the chapter.

The cause of most cases of low cortisol is inadequate secretion of ACTH by the HP system. It is a dysfunctional state, not a 'disease' state, i.e. there is usually nothing at all wrong with the adrenal glands themselves.

The cause of this HP dysfunction is unknown, although many studies have shown that it can result from extreme or prolonged stress. Stress causes ACTH to rise, which causes more cortisol and DHEA to be made. The extra cortisol and DHEA is designed to help us deal with the stress. However, this can only go on for so long. Eventually, it is thought that it can lead to HP dysfunction and lower ACTH. The adrenals also become less sensitive to the ACTH stimulation. The net effect of this is that cortisol and DHEA eventually fall.

Dysfunction of the hypothalamic-pituitary-adrenal axis (HPA axis) is thought by some doctors to be the number 1 cause of low cortisol problems.

## Other causes of low cortisol

*Genetic mutations* can also cause adrenal cortex dysfunction. Mutations can reduce the function of the enzymes needed to make cortisol, resulting in a condition known as congenital adrenal hyperplasia (CAH). Milder versions of this disorder occur in adults - where it is known as non-classical CAH. In CAH, DHEAS levels are high as more ACTH is secreted to super-stimulate the cortices to make enough cortisol.

*Syndromes of cortisol resistance* exist - much like thyroid hormone resistance. Cortisol resistance may cause the effect of cortisol within the cells to be sub-optimal. In these cases, cortisol levels may appear normal but low cortisol symptoms may still be present.

Note: most doctors only view low cortisol as an issue, if the severely low levels of Addison's disease are present. Mild to moderate low cortisol problems are far more common than the severe cortisol insufficiency of Addison's disease.

### My use of the term 'hypocortisolism' versus 'low cortisol'

Having discussed the adrenal glands and cortisol, I now need to be more precise about low cortisol. It should be clear from what has already been said in this chapter that low cortisol is better defined as the sub-optimal effect of cortisol within some or all of the cells. This definition includes all the possible causes, e.g. HP dysfunction, adrenal gland disease and even cortisol resistance. It includes everything that stops cortisol from optimally operating within the cells. Some of the issues that result in hypocortisolism may not be visible on any current medical test. This definition is similar to the definition of hypothyroidism in the previous chapter.

So, from now on in this book, I will use the term *hypocortisolism to describe the sub-optimal effect of cortisol within some or all of the cells*. It is a more precise definition and is far less ambiguous than low cortisol.

### SYMPTOMS OF HYPOCORTISOLISM AND LOW ALDOSTERONE

Some doctors describe hypocortisolism and low aldosterone as 'partial adrenal insufficiency'. I find the term to be unclear about which hormone is being described. It also tends to imply the adrenal glands are the source of the problem - which they usually are not. Consequently, I will be using hypocortisolism and low aldosterone - which are far more specific.

### Some of the main symptoms of hypocortisolism include:

| | |
|---|---|
| Low blood sugar - dizziness, unwell, hunger | Severe fatigue, tiredness |
| Dizziness (even when sitting down) | Low blood pressure |
| Intolerance to even low dose thyroid medication | Poor response to thyroid treatment or dose raises |
| Anxiety or inability to cope with stress | Irritability or anger or panic feelings |
| Feeling cold/low body temperature | Fluctuating body temperature |
| Aches and pains | Pale skin or slight darkening of the skin |
| Skin appears thinner | Digestive upsets - may include diarrhoea |
| Nausea | Weight loss if cortisol very low |
| Worsening allergies | Trembling, shakiness or jittery/hyper feeling |
| Rapid heartbeat especially after thyroid meds | Difficulty sleeping |
| Flu-like symptoms | Dark rings under the eyes |
| Low back pain (where adrenal glands are) | Worsening symptoms in presence of stress |
| Clumsiness | Fatigue in the morning but better in the evening |

**Some of the main symptoms of low aldosterone include:**

| | |
|---|---|
| Low blood pressure | Postural hypotension (lower BP on standing) |
| Craving for salty foods | Thirst |
| Light headedness on standing | Frequent urination (esp. during the night) |
| Excessive sweating | Slightly higher body temperature than usual |
| High heart rate/palpitations | Cognitive fuzziness |
| Dizziness or fainting | Low sodium and high potassium |

Note: low aldosterone can occur with or without Addison's disease. It can also occur with or without hypocortisolism. So, your doctor should be aware of this and be on the lookout for any tell tale indications of it, even if you do not have Addison's disease.

**Low levels of thyroid hormone can cause several symptoms of hypocortisolism**

This can obviously make recognising hypocortisolism a bit of a challenge. If someone has been hypothyroid for a considerable time before diagnosis and treatment, it is possible that there will be hypocortisolism present. Therefore, hypocortisolism is something that a family doctor or endocrinologist should either check for, or at the very least, be on the lookout for.

**Summary of the main causes of hypocortisolism:**

- Hypothalamic-pituitary (HP) dysfunction (perhaps due to prolonged or severe stress).
- Autoimmune disease of the adrenal glands. This can eventually become more severe and lead to Addison's disease.
- Central adrenal insufficiency. This means that one or both of the pituitary or hypothalamus glands are diseased or damaged.
- Low adrenal or low thyroid hormones after a woman gives birth - this is quite common, but it often corrects itself after a few months.
- Hypothyroidism.
- Low sex hormones, e.g. in peri-menopause or post-menopause, if they induce HP dysfunction (see Chapter 21).
- High oestrogen (which counteracts cortisol-effect in the tissues).
- A severe vitamin or mineral deficiency (which can also occur after childbirth).
- If someone has been taking HC for a prolonged period of time, the HPA-axis can be suppressed and take months to recover if the adrenal medication is eventually reduced or withdrawn.
- Environmental toxins that are interfering with cortisol production.
- Genetic defects affecting the enzymes involved in cortisol production within the adrenals.
- Cortisol resistance within the cells. This can cause hypocortisolism symptoms when cortisol test results look normal.

### Hypocortisolism may be exposed during thyroid treatment

After someone has been hypothyroid for some time, when thyroid treatment starts, hypocortisolism problems can show up. Thyroid hormone replacement may not correct the symptoms. Body temperature may remain low or fluctuate up and down during the day. If cortisol is very low, rapid heart rate and anxiety may occur (often because the adrenals produce more adrenaline, in order to continue to keep glucose levels up in the bloodstream).

If you feel much worse on thyroid treatment, hypocortisolism may be a likely cause. Raising T3 in the cells increases the demand for cortisol. Thyroid treatment can make hypocortisolism worse, e.g. worse fatigue, achiness, brain fog etc. On the other hand, increasing the T3 level can improve cortisol secretion and in some cases treat hypocortisolism. I have discussed this in *Recovering with T3* and *The CT3M Handbook*.

### Hypocortisolism can be confusing

If hypocortisolism problems persist, it is possible that the patient's thyroid blood test results will look normal but they still feel ill. Consequently, if the doctor is using only thyroid blood tests and does not spot the cortisol issue, the individual may never fully recover.

## TREATMENT OPTIONS FOR HYPOCORTISOLISM (WHEN ADDISON'S HAS BEEN EXCLUDED)

It is immensely sensible to do testing of cortisol level up-front, prior to thyroid treatment. If cortisol is tested prior to any thyroid treatment begins, hypocortisolism can be detected.

If the hypocortisolism is mild, the approach that is probably the most common is to just begin thyroid treatment. This can work. If the patient is on the right thyroid treatment for them, the hypocortisolism may resolve.

If the test results show moderate hypocortisolism, some form of cortisol treatment might be administered, before starting thyroid medication. It would be advisable to be guided by an experienced specialist in this. However, if there were no Addison's disease or low aldosterone, even very low cortisol would not be dangerous if thyroid hormone were administered. It might make you feel a lot worse, but it would not be a severe risk as long as the adrenal glands themselves are healthy.

Alternatively, even in the situation of moderate hypocortisolism; thyroid treatment could be started and be monitored carefully. Often cortisol improves with the right thyroid treatment. This is because the hypocortisolism exists in many cases due to low thyroid hormone.

It is also common for doctors to administer thyroid treatment and just try to see if tell tale signs of hypocortisolism appear. If they do, laboratory tests for cortisol might be done at that point.

Various treatments are possible if cortisol is low. Sometimes small, physiological doses of adrenal glandulars or hydrocortisone (HC) are given. These can help to raise a patient's cortisol enough to reduce the symptoms. If this approach is taken, when the patient is on the right dosage of thyroid hormone, the adrenal support may be reduced, tapering it to zero.

Note - HC is identical to human cortisol. HC also has some aldosterone-effect. Patients on HC usually need less fludrocortisone as a result of this. People who require HC often carry stress doses with them, and some wear medical alert jewellery.

If HC is used for a long time, it will reduce the body's ability to make its own cortisol. This is usually reversible, but it can take weeks or months if the HC is weaned.

*Once on HC medication*, it is important never to reduce it quickly. HC has some aldosterone-like effect, reducing it quickly could cause extremely low blood pressure and be dangerous. Therefore, all HC reduction should be done slowly and carefully, in order to allow time for the HP system to recover.

*If you are on HC medication*, it is also important to realise that there are situations of increased physical or emotional stress, which will require you to increase the HC, e.g. more physical work or a fever. Your doctor should have fully acquainted you with this information.

I will discuss the diagnosis and treatment of hypocortisolism and the risks associated with it further in Chapter 11.

In the treatment chapters, I will discuss the Circadian T3 Method (CT3M), which I wrote about in my first two books. This is an approach that does not require HC or adrenal glandulars in order to raise cortisol levels over the day in some people.

## SYMPTOMS OF EXCESS ADRENAL HORMONES

**These are some of the clues when high cortisol is present:**

| | |
|---|---|
| High blood pressure | Bruising easily |
| Fluid retention | Weight gain, obesity, or moon-shaped face |
| Increased belly fat, fat on back of the neck | Fatigue |
| Weak muscles and muscle loss | Facial flushing |
| Bile acid indigestion - burning in stomach | Mood swings - anxiety, depression, irritability |
| Reduced TSH | Reduced FT3, increased rT3 |

**These are some of the clues when high aldosterone is present:**

| | |
|---|---|
| High blood pressure | Low potassium (weakness/muscle spasms) |
| Numbness or tingling in the extremities | Frequent urination |

Please ask your doctor to run lab tests for cortisol and/or aldosterone if you suspect excess adrenal hormones.

## LIST OF ADRENAL DIAGNOSES FOR BACKGROUND INFO

The following are established adrenal diagnoses. I list them because they may be the only medical diagnoses that your doctor may acknowledge. Note: they all relate entirely to the low or high production of adrenal hormones, usually through suspected damage or disease of a gland. None of them include intracellular issues with cortisol, or milder HPA axis dysfunction.

Hence, these are here for reference:

- *Partial adrenal insufficiency* - this is a type of adrenal disorder where there is less cortisol than normal for some or most of the time. It usually worsens with stress or activity. http://www.goodhormonehealth.com/adrenal-cecils.pdf

- *Addison's disease/primary adrenal insufficiency* - Addison's disease is an autoimmune disease that causes the gradual destruction of the adrenal glands. This results in low levels of cortisol and aldosterone:
  http://www.nlm.nih.gov/medlineplus/ency/article/000378.htm

- *Central adrenal insufficiency* - this occurs if the body cannot make enough ACTH. So, the adrenals themselves may be working fine, but the pituitary cannot signal the adrenal glands to produce the correct amounts of cortisol. Central adrenal insufficiency is said to be more common than primary adrenal insufficiency.

- *Cushing's syndrome* - this is a disorder caused by prolonged exposure to high levels of cortisol. It is generally the result of a tumour of some kind or by long-term usage of very high doses of HC or prednisolone. There is also a form of Cushing's called Cyclical Cushing's that causes a person to swing from high levels of cortisol to normal levels of cortisol. http://www.nlm.nih.gov/medlineplus/ency/article/000348.htm

- *Congenital adrenal hyperplasia (CAH)* - this is a genetic mutation involving a defect in the enzymes needed to produce cortisol. As a result, the adrenal glands are constantly stimulated in a desperate attempt to make cortisol. Since the adrenal glands also make androgens, this can result in large amounts of testosterone going into the blood stream. The adrenals also produce too much DHEA - which is converted into testosterone. DHEA counteracts cortisol strongly, so much so that a person can suffer from hypocortisolism at the tissue level, in the face of mid-range cortisol levels. This disorder is almost always diagnosed at birth as it results in virilisation (masculinization) of female genitals. https://en.wikipedia.org/wiki/Congenital_adrenal_hyperplasia

- *Late-onset congenital adrenal hyperplasia (LOCAH)* - this is a type of CAH that presents anytime from early childhood to early adulthood. Genitals appear normal at birth with this condition, but the person generally encounters problems during puberty. LOCAH is often misdiagnosed as Polycystic Ovarian Syndrome (PCOS), as it has very similar symptoms:
http://www.fertstert.org/article/S0015-0282(16)59339-X/pdf

This chapter should have provided you with enough background knowledge on the role of the adrenals within our energy system.

## RESOURCES

Here is a list of further reading for those who wish to gather more background on the adrenal glands and hypocortisolism:

1. ***Addison's support group forum*** - See https://addisonssupport.com
2. ***Safe Uses of Cortisol*** - William McK. Jeffries
3. ***Hormone Handbook*** - Thierry Hertogue.
4. ***Steroidogenesis diagram*** - https://upload.wikimedia.org/wikipedia/commons/thumb/1/13/Steroidogenesis.svg/865px-Steroidogenesis.svg.png (shows the pathways involved in the production of cortisol, aldosterone and sex hormones).
5. ***Recognising and responding to adrenal emergencies*** - https://www.addisons.org.uk/articles.html/articles-for/emergencies/recognising-and-responding-to-adrenal-emergencies-r13/
6. ***Can LDL cholesterol be too low? Possible risks of extremely low levels*** - Olsson AG, Angelin B, Assmann G, Binder CJ, Björkhem I, Cedazo-Minguez A, Cohen J, von Eckardstein A, Farinaro E, Müller-Wieland D, Parhofer KG, Parini P, Rosenson RS, Starup-Linde J[13], Tikkanen MJ, Yvan-Charvet L.
   J Intern Med. 2017 Jun;281(6):534-553. doi: 10.1111/joim.12614.
   See: https://www.ncbi.nlm.nih.gov/pubmed/28295777

# Chapter 6

## The Mitochondria

The mitochondria are the engine in our energy system that provides energy to the cell nuclei (to spin the wheels of the car). But what exactly are they?

### THE BASICS OF THE MITOCHONDRIA

Each cell of the body contains various entities. In this chapter, the only two we are interested in are the cell nucleus and the mitochondria. Each cell in the human body has only one nucleus. However, cells vary in the number of mitochondria that they have. Liver cells for example have about 2,000 mitochondria per cell, whereas red blood cells have no mitochondria.

Almost all the DNA (genetic material) of a human cell is contained within the cell nucleus. The mitochondria have their own, independent, small genome that is similar to the genome of bacteria. Some of these genes are central to the main function of the mitochondria.

Mitochondria produce and supply energy to the cell nuclei, i.e. to all of the cells of our body. The mitochondria are the engine that drives the wheels (cell nuclei) in our car analogy. The energy they produce is in the form of a chemical called adenosine triphosphate (ATP). If ATP is low, the cells will not be able to perform their function at the right speed. This is true even if there is enough thyroid hormone, i.e. even if the accelerator/gas pedal is being pressed very hard. If the mitochondria are not working well, we will not work well either.

Dr. Sarah Myhill, is a UK-based doctor, who specialises in the treatment of Chronic Fatigue Syndrome (CFS). Dr. Myhill believes that CFS is often caused by mitochondrial dysfunction. Her arguments are convincing. See **reference 3** in Resources for more information on Dr Myhill.

Each cell has a sequence of chemical reactions involving the mitochondria. This sequence needs a number of chemicals, including oxygen and blood sugar. It results in the release of energy. The sequence of reactions is known as cell respiration.

Your thyroid hormones could be perfect but it will not make any difference if there is not enough ATP.

### What do the mitochondria need to perform their job?

For the mitochondria to work well they need all the right ingredients and co-factors. The two main fuels that the mitochondria require, in order to make ATP, are oxygen and glucose.

However, there are other co-factors that make the mitochondria work more efficiently. These are: the amino acid L-carnitine, vitamin B3, magnesium and co-enzyme Q10.

Dr. Myhill talks in her books about the value of anti-oxidants. If these are low, inflammation may result and free radicals can be prevalent. There are a number of useful anti-oxidants (Co-Q10 doubles up as one of these also).

Please see Dr Myhill's first book in Resources at the end of the chapter for more on this.

### The mitochondria are stimulated by thyroid hormone and cortisol

Research has shown that the mitochondria work faster when T3 levels or cortisol levels rise. Mitochondria are stimulated to some extent by T3 (the accelerator/gas pedal) and cortisol (the gearbox/transmission). This is another important set of links within our energy system.

### WHAT CAN GO WRONG

My focus in the *Thyroid Patient's Manual* is primarily to provide people with enough information to ensure that they can recover from hypothyroidism. If someone suspects that they have mitochondrial disease or CFS, please read the books in Resources at the end of the chapter.

In terms of the mitochondrial part of our energy system, here are just some of the things that can go wrong:

- Glucose may not flow into the cells at a sufficient rate or level. Insulin issues can cause this. Hypoglycaemia and dietary issues can also be a problem. Hypocortisolism problems can limit glucose levels, as cortisol is responsible for conserving a healthy level of glucose in the bloodstream.

- Hypocortisolism (sub-optimal cortisol-effect in the cells) and/or hypothyroidism (sub-optimal T3-effect in the cells) can also slow down the mitochondria, as cortisol and T3 both stimulate the mitochondria. If, hypothyroidism is not correctly treated, after some time, the mitochondria within the cells can reduce in number.

- Deficiencies in other key chemicals, vitamins, minerals or amino acids will hamper the mitochondria. Some of these include: oxygen (carried in the haemoglobin in red blood cells - so iron is important), L-carnitine, B3, magnesium, CoQ10.

- The lack of various anti-oxidants may cause inflammation and free radicals that induce lower mitochondrial activity.

- It is important to be aware that the body has good compensatory techniques. Once in a hypothyroid state, the body begins to try to conserve energy. In some cases, this may only manifest as mild symptoms. Even issues like low cortisol may be compensated for, at least for a while, and if the deficit is not large. So, for example, slightly lower glucose to the cells may not always immediately have a huge impact on thyroid hormone action - at least as far as someone can detect it. The impact on symptoms might be negligible. But at least you can see how the mitochondria fit in our energy system, and worst case, what might go wrong.

## DIAGNOSIS AND TREATMENT OPTIONS

If hypothyroidism or hypocortisolism is a big factor in slower mitochondrial activity, when these are resolved the mitochondrial problems should also resolve. This may take some time. Good diet, some supplements, enough sleep, the right type and level of exercise should all help that. Rectifying any gut or digestion issues may also be important.

If problems persist, it may take specialist help, as diagnosing mitochondrial disease is no simple thing. It takes an expert to know what the right tests are and how to interpret them.

There is enough information here for you to see how the mitochondria fit into our overall energy system.

## RESOURCES

Here is a list of further reading for those who wish to gather more background on the mitochondria:

1. ***Diagnosis and Treatment of Chronic Fatigue Syndrome and Myalgic Encephalitis*** - Dr Sarah Myhill. (This is a wonderful book. It covers far more than mitochondrial issues. It could be the gateway to good health for many people).
2. ***Sustainable Medicine*** - Dr Sarah Myhill (This discusses an overall package of treatment approaches for chronic fatigue and weary mitochondria).
3. ***Dr Sarah Myhill Bio*** - See: http://me-pedia.org/wiki/Sarah_Myhill

# Chapter 7

# Important Relationships Within Our Energy System

There are several important relationships between the critical parts of our energy system to be aware of during thyroid treatment.

## TSH and the conversion of T4 to T3

When T4 based thyroid treatments are used, after a dosage increase, a predictable pattern frequently occurs. An initial improvement happens after the medication has been increased. However, very often, after several days, any improvement can vanish, leaving the person feeling as if the increase never happened. This is totally explainable by the effect the increase has had on TSH, and how TSH affects the conversion rate of T4 to T3.

Increasing the medication initially raises FT4 levels. This, in turn, increases FT3, through conversion from a higher FT4. In the cases of NDT and T4/T3, there is also additional T3. However, when TSH eventually falls to a lower level (due to increase of thyroid hormones in the bloodstream), the conversion rate of FT4 to FT3 also falls. Consequently, FT3 lowers to a level similar to that present prior to the thyroid medication increase, and rT3 rises.

*A lower TSH results in worsening conversion rate from T4 to T3, i.e. lower FT3 and higher rT3.* It can take several increases, and possibly a very low, or even suppressed, TSH before a higher level of thyroid medication provides more lasting improvements in symptoms. However, for those on T4-based thyroid medication, who have other conversion issues, reduced conversion from lower TSH may prove problematic. They may never get to a balance of FT3 and FT4 that they had when they were well. It may need added T3 medication and less T4 medication to reach a more therapeutically effective balance.

The reverse is also true. *A higher TSH results in improved conversion rate from T4 to T3, i.e. higher FT3 and lower rT3.*

Both of these possibilities need to be kept in mind during treatment.

See *references 1, 2, 3 and 4* in Resources at the end of the Chapter for research studies that support these points.

## Hypothyroidism and the affect on the conversion of T4 to T3

When someone has developed hypothyroidism, the T4 to T3 conversion ratio can reduce. It is very common for thyroid patients to have lower FT3 and higher rT3, even when they are on thyroid treatment, than when they were previously healthy.

The points that I have mentioned so far in this chapter are backed up by *references 1, 2, 3 and 4* in Resources at the end of the chapter.

## Hypocortisolism

Hypocortisolism tends to cause hypothyroid symptoms. One way this can happen is through the lowering of blood sugar, which directly impacts the mitochondria. Lower mitochondrial function affects all tissues including the thyroid itself, because each cell needs enough energy from its own mitochondria.

Importantly, hypocortisolism reduces the ability of T3 to bind to the thyroid receptors within the cells, and it also reduces the effect of T3 within the cell nuclei and mitochondria.

Hypocortisolism is also part of the energy saving process when someone is hypothyroid. The lower cortisol level is created to save energy in the hypothyroid state. However, because the stress response is damped, the tolerance to energy excess and stress is much lower.

It is very common when treating hypothyroidism to find that hypocortisolism is blocking the effectiveness of the treatment. With mild-moderate hypocortisolism, thyroid treatment may be introduced slowly and the cortisol may well correct. If the hypocortisolism is more severe, some intervention may be required, e.g. with HC, before the treatment begins to work well.

In some cases, hypocortisolism can actually cause hyperthyroid-like symptoms. The adrenals are capable of making adrenaline, if cortisol is sub-optimal in the cells for whatever reason. If the adrenals compensate with adrenaline, the tell tale symptoms of anxiety, tension, jitteriness, high heart rate or a thumping heart, and a general feeling of edginess are often present. These symptoms can appear like excess thyroid hormone, or even high cortisol. Determining what is going on can sometimes be difficult without careful clinical assessment, and potentially, further lab testing.

## High cortisol

High cortisol also tends to cause hypothyroid symptoms, by reducing TSH, and lowering T4 to T3 conversion. High cortisol also raises Thyroid Binding Globulin (TBG), which tends to reduce FT3 levels thus adding to the tendency towards hypothyroidism. So, it is all too easy for a doctor to think that symptoms like fatigue and weight gain are due to the hypothyroidism, whereas they are actually due to high cortisol. However, symptoms like higher BP, facial flushing and fluid retention may provide some clues that high cortisol is present. See Chapter 5.

Note: powerful cortisol medications have been used in treating hyperthyroidism for this reason, i.e. to lower TSH. So, if you have high cortisol, this may limit the success of thyroid treatment.

In some cases, this situation can be a vicious circle. I have seen people who have been on T4 or NDT treatment with poor conversion. When low FT3 and high rT3 is present, this can actually raise cortisol - perhaps due to stress on the body. I have seen high cortisol normalise when the person began using T3-Only treatment, perhaps due to lower rT3.

## Hypothyroidism, hypocortisolism, and the mitochondria

T3 and cortisol both make the mitochondria work more efficiently. Hypothyroidism or hypocortisolism slows down the mitochondria. Not knowing what the FT3 level is, and not testing cortisol properly, can therefore be a cause of missing the real reason that someone is not improving on thyroid treatment.

## T3 thyroid hormone and cortisol

T3 and cortisol act together to make us feel and function well. T3-effect and cortisol-effect within the cells must be sufficient and in balance. Together these two hormones largely determine our mental and physical energy and stamina. Deficiencies of one or both of these hormones lowers metabolic rate, which causes many symptoms, e.g. fatigue, achiness and cognitive dysfunction. We require sufficient cortisol to cope with the stress of life; without sufficient cortisol we become mentally and physically disabled and prone to allergies and autoimmune disease.

T3 and cortisol have powerful interactions. Sufficient cortisol is needed for T3 to be effective within the cells. Cortisol also enhances the ability for enough T3 to bind to the thyroid receptors. T3 stimulates ACTH/cortisol secretion. T3 increases cortisol utilisation and metabolism. *T3 and cortisol work in unison.*

More T3 may make hypocortisolism better or worse. Too much cortisol reduces TSH and T4 to T3 conversion. For some, simply switching to T3-Only, or T3-Mostly, or NDT treatment, can resolve hypocortisolism. T3 itself can act as a stimulant to the HPA axis and adrenals to help produce more cortisol. However, using T3-containing thyroid medication does not work in all cases.

Thyroid hormones can sometimes lower cortisol. As any thyroid medication type is increased, more cortisol will be needed. If there is some dysfunction in the HPA axis or with the adrenals, levels will fall. Thus, in this situation, the increase in thyroid medication can make you feel worse rather than better.

*When thyroid hormone issues are being treated, it is clearly essential to consider cortisol at the same time.*

## The 24-hour circadian relationship of TSH, FT4, FT3 and cortisol

Cortisol has a distinct rhythm over 24-hours. Most healthy people have a similar circadian rhythm. 3-4 hours before getting up in the morning, our cortisol levels begin to rise. Our cortisol levels are highest soon after waking in the morning. It seems that we need to start our days *tanked-up* with cortisol. From that morning peak, cortisol levels fall throughout the day. Cortisol levels are quite low from early evening until around 2-3 hours after falling asleep. Then the production of cortisol begins to rise again.

Thyroid hormone also has a circadian rhythm. TSH peaks around midnight for most people, and FT3 peaks a few hours later. As FT3 begins to rise, FT4 begins to fall. Why is this?

Surely, when TSH is far higher, the thyroid should be producing more T4 as well as T3, i.e. FT4 should also rise?

This is because the conversion rate of FT4 to FT3 increases, as TSH rises, i.e. more FT4 is consumed and converted to FT3.

These graphs come directly from the research article: *Free Triiodothyronine Has a Distinct Circadian Rhythm That Is Delayed but Parallels Thyrotropin Levels* by W. Russell, R. F. Harrison, N. Smith, K. Darzy, S. Shalet, A. P. Weetman, and R. J. Ross. The dotted line is the mean hormone level at a given time, and the solid line is a prediction based on masses of data (the pattern is obvious regardless of which line you look at):

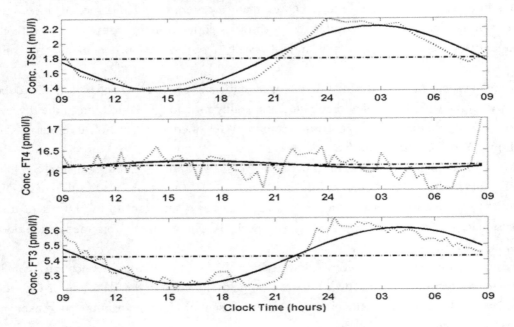

This graph is simpler but illustrates the circadian rhythm of cortisol. It comes from: http://www.endocrinesurgeon.co.uk/index.php/adrenals-the-cortex-cortisol:

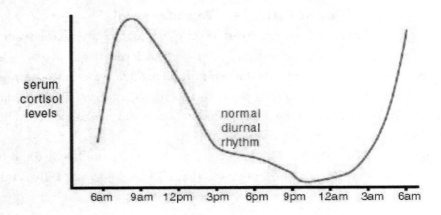

These relationships seem obvious to me now, although I have heard no one else discuss them. Current practices for thyroid treatment make no allowance for these relationships.

It is essential that the body is fully loaded up to a healthy peak FT3 level before the adrenal glands launch into the biggest drive of the 24-hour cycle to make cortisol. T3 energises the hypothalamic-pituitary system to make more ACTH, to stimulate the adrenals. The pituitary normally has the highest concentration of T3 out of all organs and glands. So, I believe that a good T3 level is needed to help the HP system drive this morning cortisol surge.

In healthy people, without thyroid or adrenal issues, the night-time T3 rise contributes to the early-morning rise in cortisol levels. The 24-hour circadian rhythms of the thyroid and cortisol systems are related. It is essential for a normal, healthy start to the day that cortisol rises to its daily peak at about the time we wake up, i.e. that we are fuelled with cortisol when we wake. So, this rise in T3 level in the night is important for good health!

Anything that lowers T3 levels in the HP system can impact ACTH, and, therefore, cortisol, e.g. a conversion issue, or simply daytime dosing of thyroid medication in some people.

I have been using the knowledge of the circadian rhythms of T3 and cortisol, and the relationship between them, for about 10 years, when helping thyroid patients. It is important.

## The Circadian T3 Method (CT3M) and cortisol

I created CT3M to increase my own cortisol levels on waking and over the day. In essence, CT3M involves taking a dose of T3 several hours before getting up in the morning. I will discuss more of the details of CT3M in Chapter 18.

I have heard from many people who have recovered from hypocortisolism using CT3M. My own cortisol levels prior to using CT3M were so awfully low that I would often pass out when I stood up, or tried to walk too far, or exerted myself too much.

Through reading endocrinology textbooks, I realised that the 24-hour circadian rhythms of TSH, the thyroid hormones and cortisol production were linked and important. The connections were not made in the textbooks, but the patterns were there, waiting to be noticed.

Using these observations, I discovered that my daily cortisol secretion improved by about 300% by taking my first T3 dose several hours before I got up. This powerful boost of morning cortisol secretion is why CT3M is a helpful tool. I went on, with the help of my doctor, to prove the connection clearly, with multiple 24-hour urinary cortisol collections, performed after different timings of my night T3 dose. T3 tends to stimulate cortisol secretion whenever it is taken, but taking a dose of T3 1.5-4 hours before rising often has the biggest impact.

## The problem with daytime-only dosing of thyroid medication

When someone is taking thyroid medication the natural cycle of thyroid hormone production does not occur. Most patients are advised to take their thyroid medication (usually T4) when they get up. Doctors have ignored the consequences of this. Daytime doses of T4 or NDT (and even T3) cannot mimic the natural circadian rise of FT3 levels in the night.

Because of the way most patients are told to take their thyroid medication, they typically have low to mid-range FT3 levels later in the day, and certainly in the night. These FT3 levels may not always support sufficient cortisol production. This is one reason that cortisol issues often begin after someone begins thyroid treatment, even though they may never have had hypocortisolism prior to the onset of hypothyroidism.

The above logic is applicable to all thyroid medication types. Daytime replacement of thyroid medication can leave many people with lower cortisol levels than they had in the past.

All thyroid medications when taken in the daytime tend *not* to reproduce a natural circadian rhythm of either thyroid hormone or cortisol. T4-monotherapy is definitely the worst, but even NDT and T3-Only can have issues when daytime-only dosing is done.

I am hopeful for a day when we can wear a device like a watch, or a patch, that delivers thyroid hormones over 24-hours, and in a natural circadian rhythm. An invention like this would resolve many issues, especially if it could be tailored for an individual in terms of the mixture of T4 and T3.

## RESOURCES

Here is a list of further reading for those who wish to gather more background on the material discussed above:

1. *Regulation of Thyroidal Deiodinase Activity* - Conti, A., Studer, H., Kneubuehl, F., Kohler, See: H. Endocrinology, Vol. 102 (1):321-329, 1978.

2. *Effect of thyrotropin on conversion of T4 to T3 in perfused rat liver* - Ikeda, K., Takeuchi, T., Ito, Y., Murakami, I., Mokuda, O., Tominaga, M., Mashiba, H. See: Life Sciences, Volume 38, Issue 20:1801-1806, 1986

3. *Effect of TSH on conversion of T4 to T3 in perfused rat kidney* - Ikeda, T., Honda M., Murakami, I., Kuno, S., Mokuda, O., Tokumori, Y., Tominaga, M., Mashiba, H. See: Metabolism, Volume 34, Issue 11:1057-1060, 1985.

4. *Homeostatic equilibria between free thyroid hormones and pituitary thyrotropin are modulated by various influences including age, body mass index and treatment* - Hoermann R, Midgley JEM, Giacobino A, Eckl WA, Wahl HG, Dietrich JW, Larisch R. See: Clin Endocrinol (Oxf) (2014) 81:907–915. doi:10.1111/cen.12527

5. *Recovering with T3* - Paul Robinson (where the Circadian T3 Method was first introduced, the connection between TSH and T4 to T3 conversion is also mentioned).

6. *The CT3M Handbook* - Paul Robinson (Contains more information on correcting hypocortisolism using T3 medication).

7. *Why the Circadian T3 Method is So Important (blog post with video)* - http://recoveringwitht3.com/blog/why-circadian-t3-method-so-important-video-version - Paul Robinson. Direct YouTube link - https://www.youtube.com/watch?v=gGs6po4D-YI - Paul Robinson.

# Chapter 8

## Do You Have Hypothyroidism?

If you think that you have hypothyroidism, your symptoms are going to be very important in diagnosing it. Having a full thyroid blood test panel is also important.

### SYMPTOMS SHOULD BE THE MOST IMPORTANT ASPECT IN DIAGNOSIS

In Chapter 4 there is a table that shows most of the main symptoms that can result if an individual has hypothyroidism. Please go back and take a look through the table for a more comprehensive review of symptoms.

Here are some of the most common symptoms:

| | |
|---|---|
| Fatigue/tiredness/needing more sleep | Feeling cold/cold hands or feet |
| Low body temperature | Lower heart rate |
| Weight gain | Feeling mentally foggy |
| Constipation | Depression |
| Dry skin or hair or coarse hair | Losing outer parts of the eyebrows |
| Poor fingernail quality (brittle, cracked) | Muscle or joint pain |
| Thickening or swollen skin (myxoedema) | Mood swings |
| Impaired thinking ability (brain fog) | Poor memory |
| Lack of concentration | Swallowing problems/swollen tongue |

If you have a few of the above, you should begin to suspect hypothyroidism. If you have many of the above, definitely suspect hypothyroidism. In either case, it is time to get this investigated properly.

There are a few things that you can do at home prior to seeing your doctor.

### Body temperature

I recommend buying a good, non-electronic, oral thermometer. Geratherm are a good make and provide reliable readings.

Body temperature can provide an insight into what is happening with your metabolism. It often reveals thyroid hormone issues where thyroid blood tests have not. But it needs to be used in the right context, along with symptoms and your medical history.

The body temperature is usually taken by placing the thermometer under the tongue for at least 3 minutes. Healthy body temperatures often fall between 97.7-99.0 degrees Fahrenheit (36.5-37.2 degrees Centigrade). Note: for women who are still cycling, ovulation can increase body temperature by 0.2-0.4 degrees F (0.1-0.2 degrees C). This rise in temperature starts 12-24 hours after ovulation and usually continues for the rest of the cycle.

Hypothyroid patients tend to have lower than normal body temperatures, e.g. 1.5-3.0 degrees F lower. However, even temperatures below 98.0 degrees F (36.6 degrees C) can still suggest hypothyroidism.

People do vary of course and some people do have lower body temperatures. *So, what is really important is whether your individual body temperature is lower than it used to be*. If it is, you are likely to feel colder and be aware of this. This may only extend to your extremities, like your hands and feet.

Getting used to using body temperature now, before thyroid treatment, is extremely useful, as it should improve if your treatment begins to work well.

I would recommend taking several body temperature readings each day over a period of several days, ideally at the same times, in order to develop a clearer picture of how body temperature is varying.

There are some things that can affect your body temperature reading:
- Eating or drinking anything during the 15 minutes beforehand.
- Taking a shower or a bath during the hour beforehand.
- A cold or virus.
- Any exercise within the previous 2 hours.

### Heart rate

This needs to be resting heart rate, i.e. you have been sitting down for a little while. This can lower in hypothyroidism. So it is worth tracking.

### Blood pressure

Blood pressure in adults is thought to be ideal when at 120/80. Blood pressure over 130/85 is considered high in the UK (other countries may have different guidelines). Tracking it is important as it can rise (or lower) with hypothyroidism.

Heart rate and blood pressure are easy to track these days, with the availability of cheap, simple to use home blood pressure meters.

### Start a 'Symptoms and Signs' Log

I strongly recommend that you now begin to keep a record of everything related to your health. This can enable you to assess it yourself. *Symptoms* are observations of your health that cannot be measured, like energy level, fatigue, mood or mental clarity. *Signs* have measurements, like lab test results or body temperature. Recording the important things you observe about your health will be extremely useful.

Keeping all the laboratory test results (even if you have to argue to get the right ones done, then argue to get copies of them) will also be critical. For hormones especially, please record which lab did the testing, as comparing results from one test to another is often only useful if the same lab did the test. This is due to the variation in assays between labs. Note: an assay is the specific method that is used by the lab to perform the test.

## A FULL THYROID BLOOD TEST PANEL IS IMPORTANT BUT ONLY WHEN COUPLED WITH SYMPTOMS

A full thyroid blood test panel includes: TSH, FT4, FT3, Reverse T3 (rT3). The autoantibodies TPOAb (and TgAb, if TPOAb is negative) are generally only tested if TSH is high or FT4 and FT3 are low. However, if your doctor is happy to check the autoantibodies, this is fine too. See Chapter 4 for the explanations of these if needed. *TSH, FT4 and FT3 are the minimal core set of thyroid labs that need to be run.*

Some doctors still request an out-dated 'thyroid profile' with a 'free thyroxine index', and a 'T3 uptake'. You must make certain that your doctor is not doing this, but is getting the TSH, Free T4 and Free T3 tests suggested here.

These tests will not tell the whole story, as they have limitations, but they are extremely useful along with symptoms, signs and your medical history.

It is vital that your doctor runs the entire panel. A TSH test alone is worthless! If this is the approach your doctor is using, there is a strong possibility that something important will be missed. A normal or abnormal TSH result means nothing without symptoms, signs and at least FT3 and FT4. Consequently, I urge you to request, beg, push, and persuade your doctor to run the entire thyroid panel. In some cases, the laboratory that runs the tests may just do TSH, and not do the others if the TSH looks fine to them. So, I also urge you to ask your doctor to put something on the test form to *request that the lab runs the entire suite of thyroid tests - even if TSH is in range!*

Getting your doctor to do the above may be hard - so go armed with information. Have all your symptoms listed and tell your doctor exactly when all this started, so that they can see that there have been changes in you. If your face, hair, skin or body shape has altered, some photos of you prior to your current condition might be helpful. Be prepared to push for what you want!

Note: in some countries (including the UK) it is particularly hard to get a doctor to run an rT3 test. Frequently, a patient has to either find a private doctor or go to one of several private test laboratories. *However, rT3 can be extremely helpful in understanding what is going on*.

*Please also ask your doctor to ensure that you get a hard copy of the full set of results*. You need to get copies of test results every single time you have thyroid, vitamin, mineral or other hormone tests.

Please also keep a record of which laboratory did the tests. Assays differ between labs, especially for hormones, so comparing results is often only reliable if the same lab is involved.

It is important to start out with the right approach and keep hard copies showing the tests, the reference ranges and the units that the result are in. From now on, you need to keep all of these results so that you can refer back to them. Start now as you mean to go on.

It is far too common to find that someone rings their doctor's office for test results only to be told by front of office staff that their results were normal. In many cases, if the results are obtained some time later, they are found not to be normal at all - but simply languishing at the bottom end of a reference range (or top end in the case of TSH). When combined with history and symptoms, mid-range or low-in-range results should ring alarm bells, especially for FT3.

*The thyroid panel tests MUST ALWAYS be done in the morning prior to the first dose of thyroid medication. So, do not take any thyroid medication (if you are already on any) on the morning of the blood tests (take it immediately after the blood draw).*

In the UK the typical reference ranges for a full thyroid panel are:
- TSH:      (0.27–4.2) mIU/L
- FT4:      (12.0–22.0) pmol/L
- FT3:      (3.1–6.8) pmol/L
- RT3:      (10.0-24.0) ng/dL
- TPOAb: (< 34) IU/mL
- TgAb:    (< 40) IU/mL

In the USA the typical reference ranges for these are:
- TSH:      (0.5-4.70) µIU/mL
- FT4:      (0.8-1.8) ng/dL
- FT3:      (2.3-4.2) pg/mL or (80-180) ng/dL
- RT3:      (9.0-25) ng/mL
- TPOAb: (< 9.0) IU/mL
- TgAb:    (< 4 .0) IU/mL

Note: these ranges may vary slightly by laboratory. In some countries, or even in different labs within the same country, the units of measure or the values may be different. So, you will need to use the ranges that your own lab provide when assessing the results.

*Even if a your thyroid labs fit within the above ranges you may still have hypothyroidism! This is critical to know at the outset.*

## INTERPRETING THYROID LAB TEST RESULTS WHEN NOT ON ANY THYROID TREATMENT

If you are already taking thyroid hormone, the information in Chapter 14 may be more relevant to you.

What I present here will not match standard medical practices. However, if someone wants to get well, this information is important to be aware of:

- **TSH** - this is not a reliable measure when diagnosing hypothyroidism. A TSH above the top of the reference range is likely to suggest a thyroid issue, especially if the symptoms also suggest hypothyroidism. If it is low, this does not rule out hypothyroidism. If it is very low, and symptoms are severe, and some of the other thyroid labs look low, there could be hypothalamic-pituitary dysfunction. Someone can also have symptoms for a long time before TSH rises. About all we can say is that if the TSH is not suppressed (if it is not near zero), you are unlikely to have excess thyroid hormone. However, if it is suppressed, it does not prove there is excess thyroid hormone. Note: there are many that argue that the upper level of the TSH range is set too high. However, by the time you have read the rest of this book you may be convinced that this, in itself, is not really that important. TSH has to be used in conjunction with the other more important thyroid labs and with symptoms and history. TSH may be mildly raised in the presence of hypocortisolism.

- **Free FT4** - a low in the range FT4, combined with symptoms, can strongly suggest hypothyroidism, especially when combined with an FT3 that is low. A mid-range or higher FT4 does not exclude hypothyroidism. A below range FT4 does mean hypothyroidism, even if TSH is normal, as this would imply central hypothyroidism.

- **Free FT3** - a low or even mid-range FT3, combined with symptoms, can be enough to suggest a diagnosis of hypothyroidism. FT3 is one of the best of the thyroid lab measures, as it actually reflects the active and bioavailable (free) thyroid hormone. *FT3 has been clearly shown to be the most useful test result during levothyroxine (T4-Only) thyroid treatment, as its level corresponds to symptoms far more closely than any other thyroid lab test result* (see **reference 1** in Resources at the end of the chapter). As such, when on no thyroid treatment at all, FT3 is a better indicator of the effect of T3 in the cells than the other labs. Even then, the focus should be on your symptoms and medical history.

- **Reverse T3** - many UK and European endocrinologists have viewed rT3 as being an inactive metabolite of T4. However, research shows that rT3 is actually a T3 blocker (a brake on the action of T3), and as such is very relevant. It is still very hard to get rT3 tested in the UK and people have to get this done privately, in combination with FT3, if they wish to assess it (which is advisable). If rT3 is high in the range, or above, and FT3 only mid-range, or below, the FT4 is not converting well. This is a strong indicator of hypothyroidism, or another problem that is impacting conversion.

- **TPOAb and TgAb autoantibodies** - If TSH is raised and FT4 and FT3 levels are low, i.e. evidence of primary hypothyroidism, it is worth running the autoantibody tests. If one of these is raised above the reference range limit, it is almost certainly Hashimoto's thyroiditis and hypothyroidism. One difficulty here is that the reference ranges are significantly different in some countries, and they may also vary by laboratory. TPOAb is the most commonly raised autoantibody in Hashimoto's thyroiditis and may often be tested first. If TPOAb were negative, it would be worth testing TgAb. Unless someone knows that they have raised TPO and/or Tg autoantibodies, they will not know whether they have Hashimoto's thyroiditis. Hence, they will not know whether to expect deterioration of their thyroid gland over time, or to consider explicit measures aimed at slowing or stopping this destruction (see Izabella Wentz's book in Resources at the end of the chapter). If the patient's thyroid does continue to deteriorate, increases of thyroid medication will be needed from time to time.

### A caution on the reference ranges

The reference ranges mentioned above are based on statistics that include 95% of 'apparently healthy' people. However, these people were not screened for symptoms. So, the ranges include almost everyone. They include TSH-normal thyroid patients and we know that these people tend to have lower levels of FT3 and higher levels of FT4 than healthy people. This means that the broad population ranges of each of the thyroid hormones have been skewed by the inclusion of thyroid patient data compared to what they would have been if only healthy, non-thyroid patients had been used to construct the reference ranges. You may need to explain this to your doctor - it is significant. It means that applying the thyroid reference ranges rigidly often results in bad decision making.

### To Summarise

It is important to test FT3 because its level corresponds most closely to actual symptoms.

During initial diagnosis FT3 & FT4 are the lab results most likely to suggest low thyroid hormone levels. If they are low to mid-range, it may well suggest hypothyroidism. So, testing both of these, alongside TSH is important.

Ideally, all the thyroid labs will be tested in order to get a complete picture. TSH alone, or TSH & FT4 are not sufficient. Symptoms need to be paramount though in any diagnosis, with thyroid labs adding to the clinical picture.

Note: deiodinase mutations, and other mild/moderate forms of thyroid resistance may cause unusual TSH, FT4 or FT3 levels. So, as I have said from the early chapters, it is all about what is going on within the cells, not the bloodstream, that counts. Many thyroid patients, including myself, have known for years that thyroid test results alone are no guarantee of correct diagnosis, or of being on the right dosage of the right thyroid hormone. *'Treat the patient in front of you and not the labs' needs to become the way that suspected and diagnosed hypothyroidism is handled.*

In many cases, if there is hypothyroidism, it is desirable to establish the likely cause:
- Is it a hypothalamic-pituitary (HP) problem?
- Is it a thyroid gland failure (primary hypothyroidism)?

- Is it some form of conversion issue?
- Is it a lack of response to thyroid hormones at the cellular level (resistance of some type)?

Certainly, reaching a conclusion on the source of any hypothyroidism would be an asset prior to treatment. To do this, all the thyroid labs must be assessed. The relationships of the various lab test results should be considered. For example, a low FT4 and low TSH could indicate HP dysfunction. If the FT4 and FT3 are very low, and TSH only mildly elevated, this could mean the same. If this is mistaken for primary hypothyroidism and T4 treatment is started, the patient might end up in intensive care, because cortisol could be quite low with HP dysfunction. In this case, it is possible that T4 medication could trigger an Addisonian crisis. So, a suspected HP dysfunction problem ought to require cortisol tests to be run, and possibly follow up tests to rule out HP dysfunction. You can see how the relationships are key. Elevated TSH and low FT3 can have causes that are nothing to do with the thyroid gland itself, so looking at the whole picture is essential. *These examples hopefully provide a good argument for why the full thyroid panel needs to be run - not just TSH, or TSH and FT4!*

The lab results need to be looked at in terms of how they play together! Most critically, the symptoms and signs, and the history of the development of the problems, and other relevant medical history must be taken into account.

### Can we ever be certain of a hypothyroid problem?

If one of the autoantibodies is raised, it is likely to be Hashimoto's thyroiditis.

If TSH is above the top of the reference range, with low or mid-range FT3, there is significant risk of hypothyroidism being present. If TSH is high and FT4 is low, you can have hypothyroidism in spite of mid-range or high FT3 (due to much higher conversion of FT4).

In the case of in-range TSH and low (or even mid-range) FT3, combined with several symptoms of low thyroid hormones, it is very possible that this is hypothyroidism.

During initial diagnosis, low to mid-range FT3 & FT4 would suggest low thyroid hormones are causing the symptoms. If rT3 is high, this adds weight to the suspicion.

In all of the above cases, it would definitely be worth treating with thyroid hormone and watching the response, i.e. doing a trial at least.

### Can we rule out hypothyroidism?

In the case when TSH is within range, there are no thyroid autoantibodies, and FT3 is high in the range, with low/reasonable rT3, it would suggest that it is not hypothyroidism. Other things should usually be investigated first before considering a trial of thyroid hormone.

### Are there grey areas?

Yes, of course there are situations where the results are not clear-cut. Many doctors would probably not want to do a trial of thyroid hormone with anyone who had an in-range TSH. But even with in-range TSH, mid-range FT3, and FT4 mid-range or above, it is still possible for thyroid hormones to be responsible for symptoms.

### What if the thyroid panel results look ok?

In the case that a thyroid panel actually looks quite reasonable, this still does not exclude hypothyroidism. Thyroid blood tests can only measure what is in the bloodstream. They cannot look inside the cells, where the thyroid hormones actually work. Thyroid labs cannot reveal the health of the mitochondria. They cannot see how genetic defects, or the effect of environmental toxins etc. impact thyroid hormones (and cortisol) within the cell nuclei and mitochondria. Even a comprehensive thyroid blood panel may fail to reveal poorly functioning thyroid hormone performance inside the cells! Mark Starr explains this thoroughly in Chapter 7 of his excellent *Hypothyroidism Type 2* book.

The medical history, the presenting symptoms, some signs like body temperature, and heart rate can be far more important in reaching a diagnosis of hypothyroidism.

> **Sometimes the only useful diagnostic test is to see what the response is to treatment!** The symptoms and medical history are crucial, with thyroid labs acting in a supporting role.

### Scans may be needed if thyroid nodules or thyroid enlargement are present

If thyroid nodules or thyroid enlargement are present, your doctor needs to get this investigated. It is important! Catching conditions like thyroid cancer early is critical to a good outcome.

Imaging tests are commonly used. Ultrasound can check the consistency of tissue (but will not detect thyroid cancer). Thyroid scans using radioactive iodine can be used to evaluate what the thyroid nodules are actually doing. Fine needle aspiration and biopsy need to be used to rule out thyroid cancer.

### TRY TO AVOID PITFALLS & ROADBLOCKS

It is critical to go into your doctor's office prepared. If you do not, you may get dismissed as being depressed, lazy or needing to do more exercise. I have heard many thyroid patients tell me shocking stories like these. Have your symptoms written down. Have some notes on how this has developed over time. If you have any measurements on body temperature etc., bring these too.

Write down what you want your doctor to do - including the list of the thyroid panel tests that you would like to be done. TSH, FT4 and FT3 are the minimal set of thyroid labs you should request. These need to be asked for and possibly argued for.

Ask your doctor to put a note on the lab test request to ask the lab to do all of the tests, even if TSH is in range.

Tell your doctor that whatever the test results are, you would like a hard copy. You are entitled to them - set his expectations beforehand. Hopefully, you will not have to argue with front-office staff.

In some countries, it is hard to get rT3 tested via a doctor. You may have to accept that and get it done privately. If you go this route, companies like Genova Diagnostics (UK) and ZRT Labs (USA) offer testing, and it would be best to do FT3 and rT3 as a pair at the same time.

Before going back to your doctor, get a copy of all the results and take time to digest them. This way, you can be prepared for any discussion and be ready to argue your case for either further testing or a trial of thyroid hormone.

Many doctors are lab-test-centric and even TSH-centric. Be prepared to argue your case. If you are not successful, do not give up!

By this stage, you should be starting to feel comfortable in the driver's seat - or at least know what it feels like to be in it!

## WHAT TO DO NEXT

If you have done all the above, you should be in good shape for the next stage. You and your doctor have the evidence of symptoms, signs (measurements at home of body temperature etc.), the full thyroid blood test panel and your medical history. Your doctor will have examined you.

The most significant focus should be on symptoms. Everything else will provide more information. If hypothyroidism is suspected, or highly likely, the next chapters will provide some insight into what to do next. Please read the rest of the book (or at least Chapters 9-14) before taking part in the discussion with your doctor - forewarned is forearmed!

If your doctor does not suspect hypothyroidism, but you do suspect it, the next chapters will help. In this case, please do not give up! Life is too short to be kept ill, when it is avoidable!

## RESOURCES

Here is a list of research studies and further reading:

1. ***Symptomatic Relief is Related to Serum Free Triiodothyronine Concentrations during Follow-up in Levothyroxine-Treated Patients with Differentiated Thyroid Cancer*** - Larisch, Midgley, Dietrich and Hoermann. See: https://www.thieme-connect.de/DOI/DOI?10.1055/s-0043-125064 (This paper clearly proves that FT3 concentrations are the most important in clinical decision making, as they are most closely linked to residual hypothyroid symptoms in T4-Only (T4-monotherapy) treated patients).

2. ***Hypothyroidism Type 2*** - Mark Starr, M.D. (explains very clearly why thyroid blood tests have huge limitations).

3. ***Recovering with T3*** - Paul Robinson (useful on the problems of being able to measure the actual action of thyroid hormones within the cells. Also more details on tracking Symptoms and Signs).

4. ***Hashimoto's Thyroiditis*** - Izabella Wentz, PharmD, FASCP.

5. ***Website blog post listing research papers on flawed current diagnostic and treatment methods*** - Paul Robinson
   See: http://recoveringwitht3.com/blog/collection-research-shows-current-use-tsh-and-t4-Only-flawed

# Chapter 9

## Use Multiple Resources - Quickly!

If you have been diagnosed with hypothyroidism, this is likely to have been by your doctor. However, you may have reached this conclusion yourself after some time, frustration, and the thorough analysis of all your information, including test results. There are some things that are advisable to do at this point.

### Join at least one thyroid forum in your own country

The Internet can be a wonderful resource these days. There are numerous patient forums that are powered by specially developed website software, as well as countless forums on Facebook. I recommend that you join at least one forum in your own country and consider joining another in a different country. I say this because different countries have different diagnosis and treatment practices. It can be very helpful to have this alternative perspective.

Some forums focus on treatment with natural desiccated thyroid (NDT), or T4/T3, or T3-Only. This can be immensely helpful. You can really use the expertise and knowledge that comes from thyroid patients that have been using a particular thyroid treatment. They have usually experienced all the pitfalls and roadblocks that are likely to occur. You may be able to avoid many of these by communicating with some of these patients.

I do suggest that you locate and join one immediately. Reaching out and talking to others who have been in the same situation as you is really helpful when you are frustrated and feel low. Internet searches or Facebook group searches should reveal these forums to you. Google is your friend!

### Find out if there are any local thyroid patient support groups

You may be lucky enough to discover that a thyroid patient support group exists in your area, or at least within travelling distance. An Internet search also ought to reveal this. If one does exist, give it a try! Your doctor's medical practice might also have some information on support groups. Speaking face to face with other sufferers may provide you with great support, and perhaps some new friends.

### Decide if your doctor is likely to provide enough of the right support

Your doctor will have listened to your story. They will have heard the description of your symptoms. They will have examined you. They will have ordered laboratory tests and you will have urged them to run the full thyroid panel. You may already feel confident in them at this stage, or you may not. When the lab tests come back, you should have a complete print out.

You should have looked at them, and thought about the results and your symptoms. You may have had the chance to discuss them with other thyroid patients. There ought to have been a good discussion with your doctor about the results and the rest of your history and symptoms.

You will by this stage have a reasonable amount of information on how knowledgeable and competent your doctor is, and whether you are going to get the support that you need. You will need on-going support and further lab testing. Consequently, it is critical to be working with the right person. You may have to be persuasive to get the support that you need. You may be surprised at how effective a good persuasive argument can be.

If you are pleased with your doctor, that is excellent. Some doctors are extremely good.

If you are not sure, please talk to other experienced thyroid patients - they will have a view on this, based on their own journeys.

If you are not pleased, there is an important lesson here that I can pass on, based on my own experience, and from working with countless other thyroid patients. Life is too short to remain ill for longer than absolutely necessary. I have heard too many dreadful stories from thyroid patients who have remained ill for many years, decades in some cases, unnecessarily, due to poor diagnosis and treatment. If you cannot work with your current doctor, look immediately for alternative arrangements. I suggest talking to other people about the quality of doctors in other practices in your area. I would ask thyroid patients on the forums in your own country for the names and contact details of doctors that are good, and that do comprehensive testing and offer different thyroid treatments. Please do not feel trapped and do nothing. It is your body and your health - not someone else's.

## Read Chapters 10-14 before starting any treatment

If you have been diagnosed with low thyroid hormones, you are going to need treatment. If possible, please read and act on the contents of the Chapters 10-14, prior to starting thyroid hormone treatment.

Chapters 10, 11 and 12 describe important steps that could save you a huge amount of time and frustration during treatment. Many thyroid patients have fallen into the pitfall of avoiding doing these, only later to find out that they were critical to the success of their treatment.

Chapters 13 and 14 provide you with tools and knowledge to use during treatment. They cover the tracking and interpretation of symptoms and signs, and how to interpret thyroid labs during treatment.

## Read the treatment options in Chapters 15-19

There are multiple treatments. If you can read through these chapters before selecting a thyroid treatment with your doctor that would be excellent. Some treatments work for some people but do not for others. I describe each treatment in a lot of detail and suggest when each might be more suitable.

**Buckle up!**

This journey can be tough. A few thyroid patients simply get well within months and remain well. Many struggle for a long time to get the right treatment. In the ***Recovering with T3*** book, I explain how it took me about 10 years to get well. It was a desperately hard struggle and one that had many costs associated with it. Other thyroid patients have similar stories, and in a few sad cases, these issues can go on for decades, as I have said.

However, the good news is that with books like this one and the many other good resources that are available these days, there should be far more swift and successful recoveries.

Do prepare yourself though. You may have to fight hard for what you need. If you need to enlist the help of others to do this then do so. ***Do whatever it takes!***

## RESOURCES

Here is one book that is useful to have on your bookshelf. It is very helpful when assessing if some other condition might be affecting your treatment:

1. ***Problem-Oriented Medical Diagnosis (sixth edition or later)*** - H. Harold Friedman. (This book is the only one that I use to look up information on medical problems, apart from Internet searches and actually speaking to a doctor. It is small and excellent).

# Chapter 10

## Common Issues that May Interfere with Treatment

This chapter is about doing the right things before starting treatment with thyroid hormone. Why would you want to do this rather than simply launch straight into treatment?

There are several good reasons:

1. Some vitamin and mineral deficiencies can cause many of the same symptoms as hypothyroidism. Consequently, if you do not resolve these, they will continue to confuse things during treatment.

2. Some vitamin and mineral deficiencies can actually disrupt the action of thyroid hormone within the cells and make thyroid treatment less effective. So, discovering these deficiencies and resolving them before treatment, is important.

3. The third reason for doing a few specific tests is to document the pre-treatment status of the heart, blood pressure etc. Later comparisons can then be made to see whether the thyroid treatment is making things worse or better.

Some of you may decide not to do any of the testing or investigation work that I suggest. You may think that doing it later is sufficient. It is your choice, of course, but it has the potential to confuse treatment substantially. This in turn can result in a far longer time to recover from hypothyroidism.

Note: testing for vitamin and mineral deficiencies is best carried out before any supplements are ever taken, otherwise test results become highly unreliable. Some supplements need to be stopped weeks or even months before lab testing.

*I will now discuss the vitamins and minerals that are relevant to the points above, as these are critical to test:*

### VITAMIN B12

Vitamin B12 is involved in many processes in the body. It helps to make DNA and red blood cells, and prevents us from getting anaemia. Hence, low B12 is known as B12 deficiency anaemia. B12 is also used to move oxygen and carbon dioxide around the body and is involved in energy production within our energy system. Hypothyroidism can cause low vitamin B12, which is thought to affect T4 to T3 conversion through its affect on deiodinase activity.

## Effects & symptoms of low vitamin B12

Here are some of the main symptoms if B12 is low:

| | |
|---|---|
| Extreme tiredness or fatigue | Lack of energy/lethargy |
| Being out of breath | Feeling faint |
| Headaches | Depression |
| Ringing in the ears (tinnitus) | Low appetite |
| Yellow skin | Sore tongue or mouth ulcers |
| Changes or loss of some sense of touch | Dizziness/balance issues |
| Mood changes - sometimes quite random | Tingling in extremities if advanced |

## Diagnosing low vitamin B12

There are several ways to do this. But be aware that if you have been taking vitamin B12 in the months leading up to the blood test, it can distort the test result and make it look higher than it actually is within the cells.

- *A B12 Blood Test* - typical reference range is 180-914 ng/L, or 200-1100 pg/mL. However, B12 blood tests cannot distinguish between the active form of B12 and the inactive form. So, if for some reason the active form of B12 has reduced, the test may not pick it up. For this reason alone, many competent physicians are starting to believe that at least 500 pg/mL should be the low end of the reference range for healthy B12 (if someone has not been supplementing it). Some other countries actually give patients injections of B12 if they are below this level, e.g. Japan. A good result is in the upper quartile of the reference range, or above. Anything mid-range or below would lead me to *not rule out* a low B12 issue. The bottom end of the range would be a serious concern. Remember, if you have supplemented B12 any time in the past months, the test result may be completely invalid.

- *Active B12 Blood Test (holotranscobalamin test)* - <25 pmol/L is considered deficient. 25-50 pmol/L is a grey area requiring further testing, e.g. via MMA (see later). >50 pmol/L is considered good. This test can only be obtained in some hospitals. The majority (up to 80%) of serum vitamin B12 is not bio-available. There is a poor correlation between circulatory total B12 and B12 at the tissue level. Consequently, it is possible that some vitamin B12 deficient patients might not be detected by the standard vitamin B12 laboratory test. The active vitamin B12 test is a better indicator - if you can get it. Ideally, you would like to have a result above 50 pmol/L. Note: these ranges are from UK guidelines only.

- *Intrinsic Factor* - if you do not have enough intrinsic factor, you may not absorb vitamin B12 in food, or in supplements. Because of this, someone with low intrinsic factor may develop vitamin B12 pernicious anaemia. The Intrinsic Factor Blocking

Antibody (IFBA) test can reveal whether there is a deficiency of intrinsic factor. This is an easy test for your doctor to run.

- **Homocysteine** - this is often raised even if B12 does not show up as a problem in the B12 blood test. If raised, it suggests a possible B12 issue. I will say more about homocysteine when I discuss folate.
- **Methylmalonic Acid (MMA) Test** - MMA is elevated in 90-98% of cases of B12 deficiency (even when B12 itself does not show as an issue). A result of <280 nmol/L is considered to be within the reference range for patients under age 65. This rises to <360 nmol/L for those over 65. These are UK guidelines only.

Note: if someone has low B12 and they are taking folate or folic acid supplementation, this can mask any B12 deficiency being detected through a B12 laboratory test. If a B12 supplement has been used, the effect of this can last many weeks, some say months, before a B12 test would yield valid results.

## Treatment options for low vitamin B12

The good thing about replacing B12 is that it is utterly safe. You could ingest a bucket full of B12 without any issues at all.

However, some people cannot absorb B12 when it is swallowed, and others need the right type of supplement. So, the treatment options that I have suggested, avoid the gut/digestive system.

If someone has a digestive system issue like Leaky Gut (permeability issues), this will reduce the ability to absorb many nutrients. So, identifying and addressing this through dietary changes and supplements may be necessary.

Low B12 can have serious consequences. If B12 is very low, it can lead to **permanent nerve damage** affecting the person concerned in many different ways. For example, it can affect the sense of touch, muscle control and even brain function. It is extremely important to detect it, and treat it properly, as soon as possible.

For the latter reason my recommendation is to pick one, or ideally two, of these treatments, depending on how low B12 is. The first two use only the active forms of B12 (so we do not have to worry about the conversion from the inactive to the active form):

- **B12 skin patches** - 5000 mcg methyl-cobalamin patches are readily available now and these avoid the digestive tract. These can be applied once or twice a week (more often if B12 is very low and needs to be raised quickly in the first weeks).
- **Sublingual Methyl-Cobalamin** - 5000 mcg/day. This needs to be held under the tongue and left to dissolve slowly and absorb through the mouth tissues.
- **B12 injections** - you can get these from your doctor, or you can be prescribed them for you to self inject (as some patients do).
- **Note** - some people with methylation pathway issues need to start lower than these dosages. I will discuss methylation a little later on. However, if you feel worse after

taking the B12, start again with 1000 mcg of methyl-cobalamin every 2-3 days and only take it more often, or increase it, slowly from that point.

***B12 needs to get treated properly if it is not high up the reference range.*** Do not let any doctor stop you from having B12 evaluated and treated if needed. Both of the first supplements I mentioned are available via the Internet.

***Note: and this is critical*** - once on treatment for B12, further testing is pointless, as B12 in the blood test may show high, even if you stop supplementing for weeks. If a doctor tests it, and it is high, he may well tell you to stop supplementing. Stopping supplementation could be a disaster! Fortunately, B12 is non-toxic, so continuing to take B12 supplements is very safe.

## FOLATE

Folate is also known as vitamin B9. It is used in the making of DNA.

It is also important in the methylation process in the body and in how amino acids are processed. Methylation is a process that creates an important protein called methionine. The methylation process creates homocysteine as a bi-product. Folate is used to detoxify homocysteine. So when folate is low, homocysteine can be high.

Hypothyroidism can cause low folate. Folate works hand in hand with B12.

### Effects & symptoms of low folate

Here are some of the main symptoms if folate is low:

| Symptoms like anaemia - same as low B12 | Reduced sense of taste |
| Diarrhoea | Numbness or tingling in the feet or hands |
| Muscle weakness | Depression |

### Diagnosing low folate

***A Folate Blood Test*** will reveal folate levels. Someone must not have been taking methyl-folate or folic acid in the 2 weeks prior to having this blood test.

The reference range in adults for folate is: 2-20 ng/mL, or 4.5-45.3 nmol/L. Interestingly, there are cases of reported folate deficiency anaemia when folate test results were in the middle of these reference ranges.

Ideally, folate should be in the upper quartile of the reference range or above. Mid-range and below is a concern and very low in the range is a serious concern - much like B12.

### Treatment options for low folate

I always recommend L-methyl-folate (rather than folic acid). L-methyl-folate is also known as L-5-methyltratrahydrofolate. For simplicity from now on, I will just refer to the optimal supplement as methyl-folate, or simply folate. Methyl-folate (much like methyl-cobalamin - B12) is easier to utilise for some patients because it is the active form. Some patients have a gene defect that affects the MTHFR gene, which prevents the use of inactivated folate and B12.

The normal suggested replacement dosage for folate is 400 mcg/day. It can go higher but the folate level will need to be retested to assess if the dosage needs to be raised. Ideally, folate needs to be in the upper quartile of the reference range. Unlike B12, you can take too much folate.

If someone had methylation issues and they felt worse after taking folate at this level, 400 mcg once a week might be a better starting point.

As with B12, if you have digestive system issues, this can affect absorption of all nutrients including folate. In this case, finding ways to supplement that bypass the digestive system is important, whilst attempting to correct any gut/absorption issues.

## VITAMIN D

When you get enough sunlight the body should make its own vitamin D. Whether vitamin D is produced from sunlight, or is obtained from a few foods, or supplements, it is then converted in the body to activated vitamin D (a hormone), also called calcitriol. When vitamin D is supplemented, it is taken in the form of vitamin D3.

Vitamin D helps the absorption of calcium - vital for bones and teeth. Vitamin D also modulates neuromuscular function, reduces inflammation and influences the action of many genes.

Research carried out many years ago, began to mention links between low levels of vitamin D and hypothyroidism. There are strong connections between hypothyroidism, autoimmune diseases and low vitamin D.

There may be several reasons why vitamin D might be low. A leaky gut and genetic defects (polymorphisms) are thought to be the two main causes.

### Effects & symptoms of low vitamin D

Here are the main symptoms of low vitamin D:

| | |
|---|---|
| Fatigue/tiredness | Bone loss/bone pain |
| Depression | Muscle pain/muscle weakness |
| Frequent infections | Hair loss |
| Vascular diseases | Arrhythmia (abnormal heartbeats) |
| Seasonal affected disorder (SAD) | Chronic fatigue |
| Osteoporosis | Serious diseases e.g. MS & some cancers |

## Diagnosing low vitamin D

Low vitamin D is diagnosed with a **Vitamin D Blood Test**. However, if you have been supplementing vitamin D recently, the blood levels may well be inflated and not represent cellular levels. Being off any vitamin D3 supplementation for **several weeks** prior to the vitamin D blood test is advisable.

The Vitamin D Council has guidelines on the ranges for vitamin D when measured in blood in both ng/ml and nmol/L.

- The ideal range:     40-50 ng/ml (100-125 nmol/L) - upper limit not to be exceeded
- Not quite sufficient: 30-40 ng/ml (75-100 nmol/L)
- Insufficient:         20-30 ng/ml (50-75 nmol/L)
- Deficient:            10-20 ng/ml (25-50 nmol/L)
- Severely deficient:    0-10 ng/ml (0-25 nmol/L)

Warning: Vitamin D assays are sometimes unreliable, and can give false results. So it may be sensible to measure vitamin D together with serum calcium, phosphate and intact parathyroid hormone (iPTH).

If the iPTH is elevated and the calcium relatively low, but the vitamin D measurement is within the range, you know the vitamin D result is false. In this case, the vitamin D test should be run with a more reliable assay (and hopefully find the true level). If phosphate is low and calcium relatively high it might indicate hyperparathyroidism (in which case, care needs to be taken with vitamin D supplementation). Testing the above ensures that compensatory vitamin D deficiency in primary hyperparathyroidism is not missed.

## Treatment options for low vitamin D

Vitamin D is usually best treated by taking vitamin D3. The Vitamin D Council recommends 5000 IUs of vitamin D3 as being very safe for adults to take daily. If someone is severely deficient, 10,000 IUs may be taken for a few months before re-testing. Larger people may need to take 6,000 IUs daily rather than 5,000 IUs based on research.

However, if you take vitamin D supplementation of 5000 IUs, or more, retesting vitamin D after 3-6 months is essential, as you do **not** want to exceed the upper limit of the ideal range.

Once within the ideal range, the supplementation should be lowered, to a maintenance dose of between 1000 and 2000 IUs.

Vitamin D3 requires some co-factors to help absorption. Magnesium is one of these, so a magnesium supplement is good idea.

Notes:

- If a patient has kidney disease, they lose the ability to activate vitamin D, so supplementation can cause more problems. In this case, it is advisable not to supplement. Discuss this situation with your doctor if you have kidney disease.
- Pregnant or lactating women are advised not to use vitamin D supplements. Consult your doctor if this is you.

- A vitamin D overdose can be toxic and cause adverse symptoms. So, if you begin to feel nausea, or vomit or experience any other worrying symptoms, talk to your doctor (looking up the full list of symptoms via the Internet would be a good idea). Very high doses of vitamin D taken for too long can cause kidney damage that is irreversible. So, following sensible guidelines is important. If there is any evidence of having taken too much vitamin D, stopping the supplementation and restricting calcium intake should be the course of action, as well as talking to your doctor.

- There is some evidence that high levels of vitamin D3 supplementation can lower magnesium and potassium. I personally know of thyroid patients, whose magnesium has dropped to an unhealthy level, as a result of supplementing with 5,000 IUs of vitamin D3 for a couple of years. I have also read articles on the Internet, written by doctors, who believe that high levels of vitamin D3 supplementation can lower potassium, thus causing an electrolyte imbalance. On the positive side, there is increasing evidence that raising your magnesium intake can help to bring up the vitamin D level - *see reference 3* in Resources. Some people suspect this latter approach is a better one for raising vitamin D, as many people are deficient in magnesium anyway. It also avoids any risk of lowering potassium and magnesium through vitamin D supplementation. However, more research is required.

An alternative approach to vitamin D supplementation is to ensure that you get out in the sun in the warmer and sunnier months. In the darker months, the use of full spectrum lighting could avoid any low vitamin D issue - light bulbs, and light lamps are available that do this.

**IRON**

Iron is a trace mineral that is used to make haemoglobin, which carries oxygen around the body. It is involved in the processes that move oxygen and carbon dioxide in and out of our cells. Iron also forms part of numerous enzymes and it is critical for energy production in the body.

Low levels of iron in the body are often associated with hypothyroidism. This is probably because hypothyroidism reduces the efficiency of absorption of nutrients in the gastrointestinal tract, leading to depleted iron levels. This, in turn, can result in iron deficiency anaemia. Without enough iron, the metabolic activity within the cells will reduce. Iron is also used by the thyroid in its production of thyroid hormones, and in the biochemical processes leading to the use of thyroid hormones within our cells. In particular, it appears that iron has a role in the conversion of T4 to T3.

**Effects & symptoms of low iron**

The symptoms of low iron may include:

| | |
|---|---|
| General malaise | Tiredness |
| Drowsiness | Dizziness/fainting |
| Shortness of breath, air hunger | Heart palpitations/faster heart rate |
| Chest pain/angina | Headaches |
| Brain fog | Ringing in the ears, tinnitus |
| Irritability | Depression |
| Anxiety or panic attacks | Pale skin |
| Pale nail beds | Food cravings |
| Low sex drive | Burning sensations in tongue |
| Dry mouth/throat/problems swallowing | Altered sense of touch |

These symptoms can easily be misinterpreted as hypothyroidism. As a result, the low iron level may be missed.

Low iron levels may also be caused by low stomach acidity that is often present in a patient with hypothyroidism. Iron is absorbed in the duodenum (the first part of the small intestine). Consequently, any condition that disrupts the health of the small intestine may have an impact on iron levels.

**Diagnosing low iron**

Thyroid hormone replacement therapy cannot succeed without an adequate level of iron. It is very important for thyroid patients to have the right laboratory tests done in order to detect any potential iron issues.

No iron supplementation should be taken for at least 7 days prior to the iron tests, apart from ferritin for which there is no need to stop supplementing.

Iron should be measured by the following comprehensive laboratory tests:

- ***Complete Blood Count (CBC)*** - this is the first test that is used to diagnose anaemia. It measures the haemoglobin and haemocrit levels. Haemoglobin is an iron-rich protein in red blood cells that carries oxygen to the body. Haemocrit is a measure of how much space red blood cells take up in the blood. If either the haemoglobin or haemocrit are low, this may be a sign of anaemia.

- ***Serum Ferritin - this may be one of the most important iron lab tests to have run***. Ferritin is a protein that is used to store iron within the tissues and it enables the steady release of iron that our cells require. Thus ferritin is crucial within the cells of our energy system. Ferritin is also thought to be involved in the conversion of FT4 to FT3 within the cells. The serum ferritin blood test measures how much storage iron is available. ***Ferritin is by far the better test of whole-body iron stores***. It is even more insightful to measure ferritin than serum iron. However, testing the full iron panel provides the best view of the overall iron situation. There is no need to stop supplementing with iron prior to testing ferritin.

Typical laboratory reference ranges for serum ferritin are 22-320 ng/mL for men/post-menopausal women and 10-290 ng/mL for pre-menopausal women. However, most female thyroid patients report that their **ferritin needs to be at least in the 80-100 ng/mL range**, which is considerably higher than the lower reference range of most laboratories. Male thyroid patients do well with similar results, or even a little higher. Ferritin below 50 ng/mL causes fatigue that resolves with iron therapy. Ferritin below 20 ng/mL causes marked fatigue and cognitive dysfunction. Low ferritin could be causing thyroid treatment problems. It may also suggest that anaemia may ensue if iron levels fall lower. A level of 50 ng/mL is considered to be 'just getting by' and iron supplementation should be considered. Note: 1 ng/ml = 1 ug/L (so no need to convert if your results are in ug/L).

However, in the case of prolonged hypothyroidism, serum ferritin may be falsely elevated, or even sometimes appear low or normal (even if serum iron is low). Inflammation can cause this. If ferritin is high, serum iron should definitely be checked. If serum iron is low or normal, and ferritin is high, inflammation is very likely. If inflammation is suspected, standard markers in the blood for this are: C-reactive protein (CRP), plasma viscosity (PV) and erythrocyte sedimentation rate (ESR). A liver function test is also recommended. Your doctor can test for these quite easily.

Note: the use of vitamin C in the ascorbic acid form is known to lower ferritin levels in some people. So, if ferritin is low, whole food vitamin C may be better to take with iron supplements. It is also worth testing ceruloplasmin, copper and zinc levels, as a zinc/copper imbalance can be the cause of low ferritin.

- **Serum Iron** - this test measures the amount of iron in the bloodstream that is bound to transferrin. This can be normal, even though the iron stores in the body are low. Consequently, other tests must also be done. Serum iron is strongly affected by recent iron ingestion, even by an iron-rich meal like red meat. Typical laboratory reference ranges for serum iron are 65-176 ug/dL (11.6-31.7 umol/L) for men and 50-170 ug/dL (9-34.4 umol/L) for women. Thyroid patients usually feel better if their serum iron is over 90 ug/dL (16.11 umol/L) and ideally close to 100-110 ug/dL (17.9-19.68 umol/L) but still remaining within the laboratory reference range. Note: ug/dL is sometimes written as mcg/dL.

- **Total Iron Binding Capacity (TIBC)** - transferrin is a protein that carries iron in the blood. TIBC measures the ability of the blood to bind iron to transferrin. In iron deficiency, the serum iron level is often low, but the TIBC is increased. In states of iron excess, the serum iron will be high but TIBC will be low/normal.

If TIBC is high, there is likely to be a low amount of transferrin not carrying iron, i.e. the ability to carry additional iron is good. If TIBC is low, the transferrin has limited capacity to bind further iron, i.e. the capacity of the blood to bind additional iron is poor.

If someone is identified as having a low iron level and a low level of TIBC is present, iron supplementation must be far lower than is normally used to avoid creating a build up of iron in the blood. In this case, the building up of iron stores will take a lot longer to accomplish, e.g. less than 20 mg of elemental iron per day may be required initially until the TIBC becomes higher. In practice, thyroid patients have found that they appear to handle iron supplementation reasonably well if their TIBC is at or above the lower quartile of the reference range.

The typical reference range for TIBC is 240-450 ug/dL. Sometimes an alternative test called the UIBC is performed. This is the unsaturated iron binding capacity and this determines the reserve capacity of transferrin, i.e. the portion of transferrin that has not yet been saturated with iron. If serum iron and UIBC are known, TIBC may be calculated as TIBC = UIBC + serum iron. The typical reference range for UIBC is 150-375 ug/dL.

- ***Transferrin Saturation %*** - this is a calculation that is expressed as a percentage. Transferrin saturation % = serum iron divided by TIBC x 100%. The transferrin saturation % tells a doctor how much of the free iron is being carried by transferrin. This is a far more useful indicator of iron status than just serum iron or TIBC alone. For instance, a transferrin saturation % of 15% means that only 15% of the free iron is bound to transferrin. Transferrin saturation % is sometimes referred to as the transferrin saturation index.

Typically the transferrin saturation % will be low if there is iron deficiency, because serum iron will be low and TIBC will be high. The typical reference range for transferrin saturation % is 15-50% for men and 12-45% for women.

The feedback I have received from experienced thyroid patients is that one should aim to maintain a transferrin saturation % in the 25%-45% range. However, recently I have read about some doctors in the USA who have found that thyroid treatment proceeds more smoothly once the patient's transferrin saturation % is in the 35%-45% range, with serum iron ideally at least 90 ug/dL. In this situation, TIBC or UIBC may be low but not actually below the lower end of the reference ranges. However, transferrin saturation % should not exceed 45%.

**Treatment options for low iron depend on the full iron panel results**

With low serum iron and low ferritin there will probably also be mid-range or high TIBC and low transferrin saturation %. This really suggests iron supplementation is a good idea. If there is low serum iron and low transferrin saturation %, but ferritin is high, this is suggestive of the presence of inflammation. In this case, iron supplementation is often not recommended until the inflammation comes down.

If iron supplementation is required, 150-200 mg daily of elemental iron is often required. This will need to be taken in 2 or 3 divided doses, as the maximum that can usually be handled at one time is 100mg of iron (if TIBC is not low). If TIBC is low, less than 20 mg of elemental iron daily may be required until the TIBC becomes higher.

If you do use iron supplements, some types are better than others for the stomach/gut. I personally prefer the glycinate or biglycinate versions, as they are easier on the digestive system. One of the side effects of iron supplements may be constipation, and so an appropriate level of magnesium in the diet may be required to alleviate this. Magnesium citrate is a good type to use, as not all types of magnesium have a laxative effect.

Iron should be taken with vitamin C (whole food vitamin C is ideal, as ascorbic acid can lower iron levels). Lactoferrin helps to improve the absorption of iron supplements. If you struggle to raise iron levels with supplementation, try lactoferrin (100 mg). If you are having hair loss from low iron, L-lysine (1000 mg) may also help.

Hypothyroid patients often produce less stomach acid than they used to when they were healthy. This can cause problems with digestion, and cause stomach upsets. It can also affect the absorption of all nutrients in the food or in supplements. If low stomach acid is an issue, taking the iron with betaine HCL may improve absorption.

It is advisable to take calcium supplements at a different time from iron supplements, because calcium may reduce the absorption of iron. Iron should also not be taken with zinc, copper, selenium, magnesium and manganese. If possible, also avoid coffee, tea and cocoa near the time that you take your iron supplement.

If you are taking thyroid hormone and iron supplements, you need to be aware of the possible interactions between these. Iron can bind to some of the thyroid hormone medication, making it ineffective. The advice is usually to take any thyroid hormone medication at least 1 hour prior to any iron supplement. Alternatively, if the iron supplement has already been taken, it is sensible to wait for 4 hours before taking the thyroid medication. Note: the same advice applies to calcium supplements, which also bind to thyroid hormone.

When supplementing with iron the full iron panel should be re-tested every 6-8 weeks to avoid iron overload.

It is also important to avoid taking iron supplements for about a week prior to any laboratory tests for iron, as this may compromise the test results. Recent findings suggest that vitamin C should also be suspended for a week prior to the iron test, as vitamin C use can also artificially inflate iron results.

## TRY TO AVOID PITFALLS & ROADBLOCKS

So many thyroid patients have gone down the road of thyroid treatment only to find months or even years later that they had a B12, folate, vitamin D or iron issue. The problems caused by deficiencies can seriously undermine thyroid treatment and stop it from working well. This can all cause years of frustration, lost jobs, difficult relationships etc. In a few cases, if the deficiency had been corrected, the patient may never have needed thyroid hormones at all.

Please get all of these tests done before you start treatment. At the very least, do them as soon as possible. Ensure that you get hard copies of the complete results and keep them safely for future comparison.

One huge potential pitfall is that doctors frequently see the test results and because they fall within the reference ranges, they are pronounced normal. We know this happens frequently. I have had first hand experience of it within my own family. I have had to get involved, to get certain things treated, when the doctor had totally missed them. Please review the results yourself. I have provided the ranges, and suggested ideals, in order to make this easier for you. Discuss them with experienced patients and get their views. Go back and push for treatment if you need to. Fortunately, much of the above can be treated at home these days, thanks to the easy availability of good quality supplements.

The above will put you in an excellent position pre-treatment.

## RESOURCES

Both of these books are good for further research:

1. *Could it be B12* - Sally M. Pacholok, R.N., B.S.N.
2. *The Vitamin D Solution* - Michael F. Holick, Ph.d., M.D.
3. *Magnesium, vitamin D status and mortality: results from US National Health and Nutrition Examination Survey (NHANES) 2001 to 2006 and NHANES III - Dai, Deng, Manson and Song.*

See:

https://www.researchgate.net/publication/256188073_Magnesium_vitamin_D_status_and_mortality_results_from_US_National_Health_and_Nutrition_Examination_Survey_NHANES_2001_to_2006_and_NHANES_III

# Chapter 11

## Test Cortisol as Soon as Possible & Compare During Treatment

In Chapter 5, I explained how important the adrenals and adrenal hormones are within our energy system. If there are problems in this area, they can totally undermine any thyroid treatment. In some thyroid patients, mild-moderate hypocortisolism can correct very quickly once thyroid treatment is underway. However, others can have much more of a struggle. Knowing whether there is hypocortisolism will provide valuable pre-treatment information.

Some of you may prefer to press straight on with treatment but I do believe, from experience, that this might end up being a poor choice. As any thyroid treatment progresses, cortisol may need to be re-tested from time to time. Thyroid treatment can place more demand for cortisol.

### A REMINDER ABOUT ADDISON'S DISEASE AND LOW ALDOSTERONE

In Chapter 5, I made it very clear that this book assumes that any suspicion of Addison's disease, or low aldosterone must be dealt with through referral to an endocrinologist. I will not refer to this again. The rest of the chapter is about testing and dealing with less serious forms of hypocortisolism.

### SYMPTOMS OF HYPOCORTISOLISM

Let me begin with a recap on the symptoms of hypocortisolism.

### EFFECTS & SYMPTOMS OF HYPOCORTISOLISM ARE

| | |
|---|---|
| Low blood sugar - dizziness, unwell, hunger | Severe fatigue/tiredness |
| Dizziness (even when sitting down) | Aches/pains, low back pain (where adrenals are) |
| Clumsiness | Poor response to thyroid treatment |
| Anxiousness or inability to cope with stress | Irritability or anger or panic feelings |
| Feeling cold/low or changing body temperature | Worsening symptoms in the presence of stress |
| Dark rings under the eyes | Pale skin or slight darkening of the skin |
| Skin appears thinner | Digestive upsets or diarrhoea |
| Nausea | Weight loss if cortisol very low |
| Worsening allergies | Trembling/shakiness or a hyper feeling |
| Rapid heartbeat or pounding | Difficulty sleeping |
| Flu-like symptoms | Low blood pressure |

## DIAGNOSING HYPOCORTISOLISM

There are various ways to do this. However, please be aware that some herbs and medications can affect cortisol testing. Adrenal glandulars and adaptogenic herbs do not tend to suppress the HPA axis for very long. So, coming off these for a month before testing cortisol should be sufficient.

HC severely suppresses the HPA axis unless the doses of HC are tiny. It has been suggested that the HPA axis can take up to 2 years to return to what it was prior to HC usage. The use of any cream product containing HC can affect the reliability of saliva tests for many weeks. Hence any cortisol testing ought to be done before HC use.

You may need to refer back to both Chapter 3 (The Hypothalamus & Pituitary) and Chapter 5 (The Adrenals & Adrenal Hormones) while reading the rest of this chapter.

*Please also be aware that hypocortisolism and high cortisol symptoms can sometimes be very similar, especially when hypocortisolism is mild. Consequently, it is very important to test cortisol to be certain of its level.*

Note: T3 is a stimulant of cortisol production. Some people never achieve a healthy level of cortisol when their FT3 is low. Understanding your cortisol level over the day can inform you about the choice of thyroid treatment that is likely to work, i.e. some people may need more T3 content in their thyroid medication, to aid cortisol production.

### Not everyone requires the same level of cortisol

Hormones, like cortisol, are not the same as vitamins. Hormone levels vary from person to person. Everyone has their own individual requirement for cortisol. Clearly, this varies over the day, but it may also vary somewhat over time, e.g. weeks, months or years. You may have a higher or lower cortisol level that someone else. This may also vary over time. It is not possible to pick fixed ideal levels and say that this is what everyone needs. It just does not work that way for cortisol.

Consequently, the following are guidelines, and as such they cannot be viewed as being fixed in stone, and the same for every person. One or more of the following tests might actually provide a clear-cut diagnosis. However, in many cases the results may be less clear. It is important that your symptoms, their severity, your signs and your medical history are all taken into account in any assessment of cortisol status.

Here are the available types of cortisol test:

- ***Cortisol Saliva Test (also known as an Adrenal Stress Test or Adrenal Saliva Test)*** - only free (unbound to protein) cortisol may pass into saliva. So, this test shows the actual levels of biologically free cortisol. ***It is the best test of free cortisol levels throughout the day and it is extremely useful during thyroid treatment.*** It can help to assess the way the thyroid treatment is affecting the adrenals and cortisol production. While it is not the definitive diagnostic test for primary or central adrenal insufficiency, it is useful in many other situations.

However, it is not always the most reliable of tests, as many things can distort the results. For example, the use of transdermal progesterone cream can cause cortisol levels in saliva to look higher. This is because the molecular structure of progesterone and cortisol are so similar. The use of progesterone cream may skew the results of some cortisol assays. ***So, backing it up with another test, like an 8:00 a.m. morning blood cortisol test is important.***

***The test usually requires four samples of cortisol:***
- One in the early morning -      ideally near the top of the reference range.
- One in the late morning -      ideally upper quartile.
- One late afternoon -      ideally mid range.
- One late in the evening -      ideally bottom of the range.

The cortisol saliva test provides information on the amount of free cortisol and the rhythm of free cortisol over the day. It also measures DHEAS (DHEA-sulfate - the test for DHEA). If DHEAS is not present on the cortisol saliva test result, it should be measured as a blood test. A low or low-in-range DHEAS, without any recent HC or DHEA use, can be a strong indicator of hypocortisolism. All of this information can be extremely useful and revealing to someone who knows how to interpret it properly. DHEA is essential to balance out the catabolic effects of cortisol in the body. A healthy DHEAS level is important.

Many times, the awakening saliva cortisol level may be fine, but it may have plummeted by noon, usually corresponding to loss of energy by then. Another example is a pattern of low morning cortisol that climbs during the day above ideal levels, which indicates that the adrenals and HPA axis are functioning but not with the normal and ideal timing. In the UK, the NHS does not offer the cortisol saliva test. However, it is easily available in the UK through companies like Genova Diagnostics. In the USA companies like ZRT offer the test. Cortisol saliva test results generally do seem to correlate well to symptoms of hypocortisolism.

I mentioned earlier in this chapter that individuals vary with respect to their hormone levels. In the case of cortisol this is definitely true. The guidelines above need to be seen in that context. There is no one set of cortisol results that everyone should trying to achieve.

Symptoms and other signs need to be assessed. A standard medical test like an 8:00 a.m. blood cortisol also needs to be run to double-check the cortisol saliva test results, especially to see if any *severe hypocortisolism* is present. If there is, further tests would need to be done, and you would need to see an endocrinologist to find the root cause of the hypocortisolism and to ensure that aldosterone was not low. *This would need to happen prior to any use of thyroid hormones.*

- *An 8:00 a.m. Morning Blood Cortisol Test* - this test needs to be performed as close to 8:00 a.m. as possible (9:00 a.m. latest). This is because the ideal morning cortisol ranges are based on blood draws at this time. Please see *reference 9* in Resources, which discusses optimal cortisol levels. I am not using the term hypocortisolism here, as this 8:00 a.m. cortisol information comes from *reference 9,* which uses different terminology.

Here is an explanation of various a.m. cortisol levels:
  - *Definitive adrenal insufficiency:*     <165 nmol/L    or    <6 ug/dL
  - *Very low cortisol levels:*     <300 nmol/L    or    <11 ug/dL
  - *Sub-optimal cortisol levels:*     <496.8 nmol/L or    <18 ug/dL

These guidelines are based on the work of endocrinologist Dr. Arlt in the UK, who specialises in adrenal issues.

- *An ACTH Short Synacthen Test (also known as an ACTH Stimulation test)* - an ACTH stimulation test measures the maximum quantity of cortisol that the adrenal glands can produce. It is the best way of identifying disease, or damage, of the adrenal glands. It is also the only officially medically recognised diagnostic test for Addison's disease. An ACTH Stim. test can also be positive in severe central hypocortisolism, as the adrenals have been without stimulation for so long that they have atrophied. The test must be done between the hours of 8:00-9:00 a.m., as all of the ideal results are based on morning readings. Do not submit to an ACTH Stim. test in the afternoon, as results may not be accurate.

An ACTH Stim. test involves:

1. A blood draw is carried out at 8:00 - 9:00 a.m. to assess cortisol (baseline cortisol).
2. Often a baseline ACTH blood level is also measured. If cortisol is low and ACTH is low, it could point to hypothalamic-pituitary (HP) dysfunction, which may need further testing.
3. Synthetic ACTH is then given, which should stimulate the adrenals to produce a lot more cortisol (if they are capable of it).
4. Further blood cortisol samples are then taken at 30 minutes and 60 minutes.

In her paper, Dr Arlt notes that adrenal insufficiency can be excluded if a person has a peak 60 minute cortisol of >600 nmol/L or >21.7 µg/dL. However, many patient advocates state that an optimal result on this test is actually at least 828 nmol/L or 30 µg/dL. Note: Dr Arlt is a consultant endocrinologist who specialises in adrenal work in the UK. She is a leader in this area. This is a test best done in a hospital that is familiar with doing the test.

An ACTH Stim. test does not exclude milder degrees of central hypocortisolism (HP dysfunction). A normal ACTH Stim. test result does not mean that an individual makes sufficient cortisol, and it does not mean that they have enough cortisol-effect within the cells. Therefore, an ACTH Stim. test. does not rule out other causes of hypocortisolism, it merely means that the adrenals themselves are capable of making cortisol and that Addison's disease is unlikely. ACTH Stim. testing on its own is not going to be sufficient to rule out hypocortisolism, as this has many possible causes, as I explained in Chapter 5.

- *An ACTH Blood Test* - an ACTH blood test is not enough information on its own; however it is useful in combination with an ACTH Stim. test, or an 8:00 a.m. morning blood cortisol test. ACTH is pulsatile so multiple specimens may need to be collected. Low in range ACTH, in combination with low cortisol, would indicate central adrenal insufficiency. High in range ACTH in combination with low cortisol would indicate primary adrenal insufficiency. Please note that ACTH specimens are highly sensitive and need to be stored on ice. Improper storage and collection of ACTH specimens can invalidate the test. This is a test best done in a hospital that is familiar with doing the test. The reference range may vary by lab.

- *An Insulin Tolerance Test* - before this test is ever done, the 8:00 a.m. morning cortisol test and the ACTH Stim. test should have been done to rule out Addison's disease, i.e. at this stage primary adrenal insufficiency is *definitely not present*. If you suspect you have central adrenal insufficiency, you may need to get this test. It involves being injected with insulin to lower your blood sugar. Then, once your blood sugar is low, cortisol levels are measured. Cortisol levels should be normal-high when a person has low blood sugar. This is because a normal hypothalamus & pituitary will work together to request the adrenals produce enough cortisol to begin to raise blood sugar. If cortisol remains low even during hypoglycaemia, this shows that there is a problem with the HPA axis. In order for the test to be valid, your blood sugar must plummet to 39.6 mg/dl (2.2 nmol/L).
See:http://www.pathology.leedsth.nhs.uk/dnn_bilm/Investigationprotocols/Pituitaryproto cols/InsulinToleranceTest.aspx
*Note: whilst this test is useful, it can also be dangerous.* It would definitely have to be done in hospital and by staff familiar with the test. If central adrenal insufficiency is present, the patient would have such low blood sugar that staff would need to be on hand to administer glucose. Because of this, it is a test that is not frequently done and might require persuasion to obtain.

- **Cortisol Binding Globulin** - this is a relatively new test that is not on most doctors' radars. However, it can be a very illuminating test. Cortisol binding globulin (CBG) is a binding protein that binds up cortisol. The more CBG a person has in their system, the less free cortisol is present to do its job. A person could have a perfect morning cortisol of 552 nmol/L or 20 µg/dL, yet all of this cortisol could be bound up by high amounts of CBG. A CBG test could reveal an underlying adrenal issue where the standard 8:00 a.m. blood test did not. Please see the following link: http://www.ncbi.nlm.nih.gov/pubmed/11834433

- **Free Cortisol Blood Test** - some laboratories can do this now. Getting this tested at 8:00 a.m., and ideally also at 4:00 p.m., would provide excellent information, if your lab can do it.

- **Home measurement of free cortisol by hand-held consumer devices** - this type of product is now in development and close to being available to consumers. I have spoken with one company that is designing such a device. The product will provide a free cortisol reading for an individual at any time and anywhere they choose to check it. It should make assessing cortisol during thyroid treatment much more practical. Sometimes, you just need to assess free cortisol in a timely manner.

Note: all the above tests focus on determining the level of cortisol, or a related hormone, in saliva or blood. They assume that everything that could go wrong with cortisol can be measured in a test. Much like thyroid hormones, this is simply not true. Intracellular issues can also exist. Hence, I have defined hypocortisolism as the sub-optimal effect of cortisol within some or all of the tissues. The above testing clearly has its place. It just may not find all cases of hypocortisolism problems. I have already made it clear in Chapter 5 that HP dysfunction accounts for the majority of cases of hypocortisolism. When the hypocortisolism is mild-moderate most of the above tests, with the exception of free cortisol based ones may not reveal anything. Even the free cortisol ones will not show any HP dysfunction or cortisol resistance.

## SYMPTOMS AND SIGNS VERSUS CORTISOL TESTING

It is important to recognise that symptoms and signs must still be the most important aspect of diagnosing hypocortisolism. Any test is capable of providing misleading results. Even cortisol saliva testing, although incredibly useful, can do this. Conditions like cortisol resistance can suggest that someone has high cortisol, yet they actually have low cortisol-effect within their cells. Some chemicals, supplements or medications can also affect cortisol saliva testing. So, more emphasis needs to be on **clinical assessment** via symptoms and signs, i.e. not a slavish reliance on lab test results alone. Please do not rely on cortisol saliva tests alone. Good old-fashioned 8:00 a.m. morning blood cortisol (or ideally free cortisol if you can get it done) is still very valuable.

## PRE THYROID TREATMENT TESTING OF CORTISOL

I have already explained that it is advisable to test certain vitamins and minerals prior to starting thyroid treatment. This definitely applies to cortisol. Understanding your cortisol status will provide you and your doctor with valuable information that will help to manage the introduction of thyroid medication. It can save you a vast amount of time during the treatment phase.

Chapter 5 listed the types of symptoms that can occur with severe Addison's disease and with other forms of hypocortisolism. Depending on the severity of your own symptoms, you and your doctor will need to decide which of the tests would be most suitable for you. *A minimal set of tests would be a cortisol saliva test (4 samples) and an 8:00 a.m. morning blood cortisol test.* If your symptoms are more severe, your doctor might wish you to see an endocrinologist in order to have more tests done, e.g. an ACTH Stim. test (short synacthen test).

*An ideal set of tests would be a cortisol saliva test (4 samples), an 8:00 a.m. morning blood cortisol, DHEAS and ACTH.* Far more information is available from this set of results. If symptoms and signs are fully assessed, other tests may not be necessary in most cases of hypocortisolism.

## TREATMENT OPTIONS FOR HYPOCORTISOLISM (NOT ADDISON'S DISEASE)

What you do next depends on which tests you have had done and what the results were. You need to discuss your results with your own doctor. Perhaps you will also need to be referred to an endocrinologist.

### Treatment of severe hypocortisolism

*This only applies in the case that your doctor or endocrinologist has ruled out Addison's disease and low aldosterone.*

The underlying cause for the hypocortisolism needs to be understood. In the cases that require cortisol replacement, the dosages required vary substantially.

HC doses over 20-30 mg can suppress the pituitary stimulation of your adrenal production of cortisol. A larger dose, used for longer than 6 weeks, will render your own cortisol production system completely unresponsive. Subsequently, if you find yourself in a very stressful situation, or have to work physically a lot harder, your system will not respond to it.

Healthy people actually can increase their cortisol level by a factor of 10 if they have to do more strenuous work, or are under severe physical stress or have a fever. If the stress response is blunted through the incorrect use of HC, in an emergency situation, people who are not on the right dosage of HC are at risk of sudden death. An emergency situation can include the sudden need to deal with large emotional or physical stress or illness/fever. In Germany, any patient who is dependent on cortisol substitution is given a cortisol tool-kit to be used in an emergency.

For all the above reasons, I have always been nervous about the free and easy nature of advice on the Internet with respect to the use of HC. Certainly, some people require HC, but I believe that tests to determine this need to be done first. Some training and advice also needs to be provided so that the individual using HC realises what to do in different situations.

In some cases, even severe hypocortisolism can improve with the use of thyroid medications that include some T3. This was my own case. My cortisol was extremely low but it improved markedly on T3-Only therapy including the CT3M protocol.

Some patients also have low aldosterone. Your doctor may feel that it is low enough to require treatment. If so, fludrocortisone (Florinef) is used to raise aldosterone levels.

## Background information on how HC is typically used

In many cases, it may be possible to correct the hypocortisolism without resorting to HC. However, here is some background information for those who want to know a little more about the use of bio-identical cortisol - HC.

Those people who work full-time, are on thyroid medication and who wish to exercise, tend to be in the 25-40 mg range of HC. Some people can get by on 20 mg; these people are not usually on thyroid meds, and do not usually work full time or follow an exercise regime.

It is important to know what a patient's DHEA level is prior to treatment with HC. DHEA needs to be at a good level in the reference range in order to stop the adverse catabolic effects of cortisol.

Two thirds of the total daily HC dosage is usually taken prior to 1:00 p.m. and the rest by 4:00-5:00 p.m. (assuming you rise around 7:00-8:00 a.m.). The dosing of HC typically starts at least an hour before rising, at lunchtime and then late afternoon. Common advice is to never take your last dose after 5 p.m. unless you have to go to bed very late, although, a few people need to take a small amount of HC at bedtime.

Typical starting doses are 20-25 mg of HC for those with Addison's disease or central adrenal insufficiency. The dosage is then titrated up or down based on results/symptoms. It is basically trial and error. Increases in HC dose (stress dosing) need to be done in demanding situations or sickness. Carrying stress doses of HC are essential, once HC treatment is in place. See *reference 10* in Resources for approaches in emergency situations.

The above dosing information is for rough background only. Please work with an endocrinologist/specialist to get any cortisol issue requiring HC or Florinef treated correctly.

Note: some patients have found that combining HC treatment with the *Circadian T3 Method (CT3M)* reduces their overall daily HC dosage.

## Treatment of mild or moderate hypocortisolism

We are in the area of sub-optimal cortisol or possibly very low cortisol (if symptoms are not severe), as described in the section on the 8:00 a.m. morning blood cortisol test.

If the hypocortisolism is causing severe symptoms, your doctor should send you to an endocrinologist who should run further tests to determine the cause. Your doctor may or may not provide treatment with HC. It would depend on the cause, the severity of the hypocortisolism and on how it is affecting you.

If the hypocortisolism is only moderate to mild, and your symptoms are not that severe, your doctor may think it is safe to commence thyroid treatment and then see how it goes.

Having had the tests done and being aware of the situation is really important though. It might also influence the type of thyroid treatment selected.

In my previous two books (***Recovering with T3*** and ***The CT3M Handbook***) I introduced the protocol that I have used myself for many years. CT3M actually corrected my own hypocortisolism, and raised my cortisol levels right across the entire day. CT3M requires no adrenal medication at all. It simply uses thyroid hormone that contains T3. Knowing that there is hypocortisolism might suggest beginning treatment with a T3 containing medication and starting with CT3M immediately, if the hypocortisolism is not too extreme and there is no underlying HP dysfunction or adrenal disease.

Note: infections (root canal, sinus, Lyme Disease, Epstein Barr etc.) can all drag down the HPA axis and cause hypocortisolism. If there is any suspicion of infection, this needs to be thoroughly investigated, as this could help to correct any hypocortisolism.

Low or out of balance sex hormones might also cause HP dysfunction (see Chapter 21). If cortisol issues persist, checking sex hormones could be essential. I have avoided suggesting that sex hormones be looked at before thyroid treatment because the process can be complex and the treatment even more so.

## A FEW WORDS ON HIGH CORTISOL

Saliva cortisol tests can occasionally be misleading in detecting high cortisol. Saliva results can certainly become falsely elevated if any cream containing HC is applied to the skin, and they can stay elevated for many weeks. Dr Henry Lindner in the USA has seen very high saliva cortisol levels in patients who swear that no HC had touched their skin in years. However, on further testing, they actually had mid-to-low serum cortisol levels, and badly needed cortisol supplementation. It is possible that the use of transdermal progesterone might cause falsely elevated cortisol results in some saliva assays (see Chapter 21). See ***reference 4*** in Resources at the end of the chapter for more information on Dr. Lindner, and ***references 5, 6 and 7*** for essays he has written, and his collection of abstracts on cortisol, DHEA and other hormones.

Consequently, if cortisol saliva test results indicate high cortisol, the best first step is to assess symptoms and signs. There are differences between the symptoms of high cortisol vs. hypocortisolism. These become more apparent when cortisol is very high or very low (they are less clear when cortisol levels are slightly sub-optimal). However, in many cases it should be possible to verify the high cortisol saliva test result by assessing the symptoms.

If symptoms are unclear, the next step is to test again but using a blood test. If your lab can test free cortisol, doing this at 8:00 a.m. (and ideally 4:00 p.m.) would be an excellent test to determine the real situation. If the test for free cortisol in serum is not available, doing a standard 8:00 a.m. blood cortisol test (and ideally testing CBG at the same time) would be the next best alternative.

If cortisol is truly excessive, for some reason, the cause of this ought to be investigated. Sometimes, low DHEA may be a factor in any high cortisol. In some of these cases, supplementation with the right amount and correct type of DHEA may address the high cortisol. I say a little more about this in Chapter 21.

Note: a low DHEAS casts doubt on the diagnosis of high cortisol, because a naturally overactive ACTH-adrenal system should also make a lot of DHEA (however, in the first instance it may be worth a trial with some DHEA). One rare exception is caused by a cortisol-producing tumour, which suppresses ACTH and DHEA production.

## TRY TO AVOID PITFALLS & ROADBLOCKS

Starting thyroid treatment without knowing cortisol status can cause many problems. Symptoms alone can be very unpleasant during thyroid treatment in the presence of hypocortisolism. I explained in Chapter 5 that adrenaline could be produced when thyroid treatment is given or increased when cortisol is low. This can be really uncomfortable!

Testing cortisol is a really good idea. Re-testing may be necessary from time to time during thyroid treatment if good progress is not being made.

## RESOURCES

Here is a list of further reading for those who wish to gather more background information on the adrenals and recovering from hypocortisolism problems:

1. *Hypothyroidism Type 2* - Mark Starr, M.D. (See Chapter 10 - Adrenal Deficiencies).
2. *Recovering with T3* - Paul Robinson. (See information on the Circadian T3 Method - CT3M).
3. *The CT3M Handbook* - Paul Robinson. (More information on CT3M).
4. *Stop the Thyroid Madness* - Janie A Bowthorpe, M.Ed. (See Addendum F - Interpreting Your Cortisol Saliva Lab Results).
5. *Dr. Henry Lindner's Bio* - http://hormonerestoration.com/aboutus.html (Dr Lindner runs his own medical practice and focuses on bio-identical hormone replacement therapy)
6. *Dr. Henry Lindner essay on cortisol* - http://www.hormonerestoration.com/Cortisol.html
7. *Dr. Henry Lindner essay on DHEA* - http://www.hormonerestoration.com/DHEA.html
8. *Dr. Henry Lindner collection of annotated abstracts on cortisol, DHEA and other hormones* - http://www.hormonerestoration.com/Evidence.html
9. *Optimal 8:00 a.m. morning blood cortisol levels* - See: http://hormonebalance.org/images/documents/Arlt%2003%20AI%20Lancet.pdf
10. *Recognising and responding to adrenal emergencies* - https://www.addisons.org.uk/articles.html/articles-for/emergencies/recognising-and-responding-to-adrenal-emergencies-r13/

# Chapter 12

## Get on a Good Basic Nutritional Supplement Regime

### WHY BOTHER WITH NUTRITIONAL SUPPLEMENTS?

I have already spent time explaining that many things can undermine treatment and recovery. Our western diet, and modern farming techniques, may also cause problems. Most people these days are deficient in one or more vitamins and minerals. People, who have been hypothyroid for some time, are likely to be more so. Hypothyroidism affects the entire body, including the ability to absorb nutrients efficiently in the gut. Consequently, ensuring that your diet is healthy is important. A daily nutritional supplement regime can complement this.

### MY APPROACH TO SUPPLEMENTS IN THIS CHAPTER

I am going to list what I think is a reasonable set of supplements, and, at the end, I will list some resources that you can use to delve deeper into this area should you wish to. I am not a qualified nutritionist, so I tend to err on the conservative side with these, i.e. there will be a limited number of them, and the dosages will be quite low compared to some other authors.

Where someone is already taking a vitamin or mineral to correct a deficiency that has already been found, please ignore the supplement in my list.

I am also not going to waste time explaining the rationale for taking each supplement. There are far more comprehensive books that already do an excellent job of this - see Resources at the end of the chapter.

### HOW TO TAKE SUPPLEMENTS

Vitamins are divided into two types:

*The fat-soluble vitamins* - these are the A, D, E and K vitamins. It is possible to take these vitamins once a day, because after they have been ingested, the body uses them as and when necessary. Ideally take these with food.

*The water-soluble vitamins* - these are the B vitamins and vitamin C. These are ingested and absorbed into the blood stream and cells, but any excess will be quickly excreted. It is therefore better to take these vitamins in small doses throughout the day, and with food for better absorption.

*The minerals* need to be taken with food.

When introducing supplements please only add one at a time and ensure that you can tolerate them.

## SUGGESTED SUPPLEMENT REGIME

If you decide to follow some of the following suggestions, please check that, if you are taking any already, you do not take excessive amounts:

- *A general multi-vitamin & mineral* - the recommended daily allowance (RDA) of most of the common vitamins and minerals is very low. This is a safety-net approach that ensures that you get at least a little of everything. I take 1 per day with food.

- *A good vitamin B complex* - 25 mg B1 (thiamin), 25 mg B2 (riboflavin - necessary for the adrenals and thyroid function), 50 mg B3 (niacin - critical to all cell function, see Chapter 6 - Mitochondria), 100 mg B5 (pantothenic acid), 25 mg B6 (ideally in the activated P-5-P form, a key for the thyroid and other processes). 45-100 mcg folate (ideally as methyl-folate). The product I am currently using also has 200 mcg of folic acid, 125 mcg of B12, 25 mg PABA and 50 mg Inositol. I take 1 per day with food.

- *Vitamin B12* - 5,000 mcg of methyl-cobalamin. The product I have happens to be a sub-lingual version but I just swallow it, as I have no absorption issues. I take 1 per day with food.

- *Vitamin C* - 1,000 mg of ascorbic acid vitamin C. I increase to 2000 or 3000 mg if I think I am coming down with a cold or infection (in which case I take them in divided doses over the day). People that have problems raising ferritin levels should consider using wholefood vitamin C, as ascorbic acid can actually harm the storage of iron in some people. Typically, 1,000 mg per day with food.

- *Vitamin D3* - If vitamin D was found to be low you will probably already be on supplementation to raise your vitamin D up to a healthy level. If your vitamin D is close to optimal, you may not require vitamin D supplementation, or if you do it will only be a low maintenance dose. I take a maintenance dose of 1,000 IUS per day with food, during the dark months of the year. See the comments in Chapter 10.

- *A Good Quality Multi-Mineral* - this has higher levels of minerals than in the multi-vitamin & mineral with which I started this list. It contains calcium 250 mg, iodine 75 ug, iron 5 mg, magnesium 125 mg, phosphorus 100 mg, zinc 5 mg, boron 1 mg, copper 0.125 mg, chromium 10 ug, manganese 5 mg, potassium 33 mg and selenium 13 ug. I take 1 per day with food.

- *Magnesium Biglycinate* - contains 250 mg magnesium per capsule. Most people are deficient in magnesium. I take 2 per day with food.

- *Selenium* - ideally chelated selenium e.g. L-selenomethionine 100-200 mcg (up to 400 mcg is permissible). I take 1 200 mcg capsule per day with food.

- *Omega 3 Fish Oil* - contains 330 mg of EPA, 220 mg of DHA. I take 1 per day with food.

- *Co-enzyme Q10 (CoQ-10)* - the Ubiquinol version is more readily absorbed. Contains 100mg Ubiquinol. I take 1 per day with food.

- *Note on Probiotics* - these are also a good idea, but do some reading up on these first. The Resources at the end of the chapter will help.

- *Note on iodine* - I do not use iodine but some people believe it is necessary for healthy thyroid function. There is much controversy over it. Deficient iodine is thought to be a factor in causing Hashimoto's thyroiditis, but excess iodine is thought to do the same! I have included a book reference about iodine below, so that you can make up your own mind.

- *Note on zinc* - if you can tolerate zinc, using a supplement may also be a good thing. Zinc is thought to be involved in the conversion of FT4 to FT3 within the cells. However, in some people, it can depress cortisol levels, at doses over 10mg. Consequently, this would have to be explored carefully, if you have hypocortisolism. Zinc can be toxic in levels above 50mg, so supplementing with 10-20 mg might be safer.

## RESOURCES

Here is a list of further reading, for those who wish to look further into nutritional supplements:

1. *Diagnosis and Treatment of Chronic Fatigue Syndrome and Myalgic Encephalitis* - Dr Sarah Myhill. (See Chapter 18 in her book - The nutritional supplements you need to recover).

2. *Hashimoto's Thyroiditis* - Izabella Wentz, PharmD, FASCP. (See Chapter 19 in her book - Supplements).

3. *The Magnesium Factor* - Mildred S. Seelig, M.D., MPH, Master, American College of Nutrition, Andrea Rosanoff, Ph.D.

4. *Transdermal Magnesium Therapy* - Mark Sircus, Ac., O.M.D.

5. *The Vitamin D Solution* - Michael F. Holick, Ph.D., M.D.

6. *Vitamin C: The Real Story* - Steve Hickey, Ph.D., Andrew W. Saul, Ph.D.

7. *Iodine Why You Need It Why You Can't Live Without It* - David Brownstein, M.D.

# Chapter 13

# Symptoms and Signs to Track During Treatment

### WHAT ARE SYMPTOMS AND SIGNS?

A *symptom* is something that a patient complains about or feels. It is a feeling or opinion, e.g. being fatigued or feeling depressed.

A *sign* is a specific measurement that someone else can observe, measure or test. One example is body temperature; another is a blood test result.

If I complained that I was feeling cold, and my body temperature reading was below normal, the sign would be the temperature measurement, the symptom would be my sensitivity to cold.

Symptoms and signs provide vital clues that can be used to assess whether a dosage change has been effective or detrimental. When a doctor talks about performing a *clinical assessment* of a patient, they are assessing current symptoms and signs, in the context of treatment and patient history.

Symptoms and signs can be used to manage dosage increases of all thyroid medications.

*The main symptoms that I have found useful include* - mood; anxiety (including restlessness and irritability); mental ability and clarity; energy level; strength or weakness; digestive symptoms; skin condition; feeling warm or cold; muscle aches and pains. You may have some others that are important to you.

*The main signs that are useful are* - resting heart rate; body temperature; resting blood pressure; weight gain or loss; blood sugar level; cortisol test results; checking that the heart is working well (no abnormal rhythms or sounds); electrocardiogram (ECG); checking for evidence of bone loss; nutritional deficiencies; thyroid blood test results.

### USEFUL DETAILS ON SYMPTOMS

- *Mood* - being down or depressed can mean that thyroid hormone dosage is still too low, or there is not enough FT3, or that rT3 is too high in relation to FT3. It can also suggest that a nutrient is low, e.g. vitamin D.

- *Anxiety* - restlessness, hyperactivity, irritability, edginess, tenseness and the inability to relax can mean too much thyroid hormone is being taken. However, it can also suggest a hypocortisolism issue, which is causing adrenaline to be produced. It can also suggest that iron, or some other nutrient, is low.

- *Mental ability and clarity* - too little thyroid hormone or low ferritin can make clear and quick thinking more difficult, and for some people, they can feel as though immersed in a thick, mental fog. Others are still able to think, but feel detached and as if under water.

- *Energy level* - general energy level and stamina tend to be good if thyroid hormone is working and properly titrated (correct dosage for the person). They are poor if the thyroid treatment is too low, or for some reason, is not working well. Fatigue during the day, and particularly in the evening, is typically a good indicator of low FT3 levels. Fatigue first thing in the morning, followed by improved energy during the day, tends to be an indicator of hypocortisolism. With good cortisol levels, the patient can wake up refreshed but can get fatigued during the day if the thyroid dosage is too low, or not working well, e.g. there is not enough FT3, or too much rT3. Cortisol might need to be retested from time to time.

- *Weakness* - this can also result from low thyroid hormones.

- *Digestive system* - the digestive system rarely lies! If thyroid hormones are low, it almost always causes constipation. This can also occur if the thyroid medication is not converting well, and there is low to mid-range FT3. The symptom would be worse if high rT3 were present too. If there is too much thyroid hormone, and it is converting well, diarrhoea can result.

- *Skin, hair and nails* - changes in the quality of these can provide reliable clues as to whether the thyroid medication dosage is optimised. However, it takes a long time for these changes to become apparent. Therefore, skin, hair and nail quality are only useful indicators after several months have passed on a new thyroid dosage.

- *Heat or cold sensitivity* - usually a good indicator, but body temperature readings are better to record (a sign), when these symptoms arise.

- *Muscle aches or pains* - I personally never experienced severe muscle aches and pains. However, I know that many hypothyroid patients do suffer from these symptoms, which may alert them to a low thyroid dosage.

## USEFUL DETAILS ON SIGNS

- *Body temperature* - I am recommending that anyone, about to embark on thyroid treatment, buy a basal thermometer to regularly measure body temperature throughout the day to see how thyroid treatment affects readings. If body temperature is around 98.3-98.6 degrees Fahrenheit (36.8-37.0 degrees Centigrade) the treatment is likely to be going well. If body temperature is below 98.0 degrees Fahrenheit (36.67 degrees Centigrade), thyroid hormones may still be too low. If body temperature is below 97.7 degrees Fahrenheit (36.5 degrees Centigrade), there is even more chance that the thyroid medication is too low.

Clearly, these are generalisations and may not apply to everyone. Some people have naturally lower body temperature. However, thyroid hormone treatment ought to raise metabolic rate, which should raise body temperature. *So, the most important thing is how body temperature changes during treatment!*

During the early stages of thyroid treatment, the way that body temperature adjusts to a thyroid hormone dose can prove very informative. As treatment progresses, body temperature should rise to what used to be normal for you.

Any exercise within the previous 2 hours can increase body temperature.

Any mild activity within the previous 15 minutes can also increase body temperature, so reclining or sitting in a room that is comfortably heated, for at least 15 minutes before taking a temperature reading is important.

Eating or drinking anything during the 15 minutes beforehand can affect the result, because it changes the temperature in the mouth.

Taking a shower or a bath during the hour beforehand can temporarily lower temperature readings.

A cold or virus can affect the body temperature - avoid taking temperature readings if a virus or other illness is suspected.

Once again, hypocortisolism problems can cloud the picture, and cause misleading temperature readings. If the adrenal glands fail to produce enough cortisol, this may have a profound effect on our energy system. If this is the case, hypocortisolism issues need to be addressed. The same comment also applies to some essential nutrients like iron, B12, folate and vitamin D.

- *Blood pressure (resting)* - I recommend that you buy a home blood pressure meter to use as you are having your thyroid medication adjusted. BP meters measure both blood pressure and heart rate. So, they serve two purposes. Only take readings when resting and relaxed. The upper arm that the BP cuff is on should be aimed away from the body (approximately at right angles to the body) and the arm should be supported on a chair arm or pillow to get an accurate result.

An individual's blood pressure is expressed as systolic over diastolic blood pressure, e.g. 120/80. The systolic blood pressure (the first number) represents the pressure in the arteries as the muscle of the heart contracts and pumps blood into them. The diastolic blood pressure (the second number) represents the pressure in the arteries as the muscle of the heart relaxes following its contraction. The range of systolic blood pressure for most healthy adults falls between 90 and 120 millimetres of mercury (mm Hg). Normal diastolic blood pressure ranges between 60 and 80 mm Hg. In older people 130/85 is common.

Current guidelines in the UK define the normal blood pressure range as lower than 130/85. Blood pressures over 130/85 are usually considered high. 120/80 or lower is ideal. Low blood pressure (hypotension), is pressure so low it causes symptoms or signs due to the low flow of blood through the arteries and veins. When the flow of blood is too low to deliver enough oxygen and nutrients to vital organs, e.g. brain, heart, and kidneys, the organs do not function normally, and may be temporarily or permanently damaged.

Anyone who has concerns should consult their doctor who will assess their blood pressure together with their other presenting symptoms.

Endocrinologists recognise that Hypothyroidism can cause raised blood pressure. Hyperthyroidism, on the other hand, does not. This is one reason why Hypothyroidism can put a strain on the heart (often lowering heart rate due to BP increases). During treatment we are particularly interested in any changes in BP.

- **Resting heart rate** - a rapid heart rate, or a feeling that your heart is pounding hard can indicate that the thyroid dosage is too high. This is one sign that I will suggest tracking well, as it is so easy to collect. This has to be checked when at rest and not within a few hours of exercise. How heart rate adjusts during treatment can be extremely insightful.

  Nevertheless, it is important to be aware that heart rate readings can sometimes provide misleading information. Taking too little thyroid medication can also put a strain on the heart, and cause an increase in heart rate. Used in isolation, the resting heart rate cannot always confirm whether a dosage is too high or too low. It is very important to use the resting heart rate, along with other symptoms and signs, before making a judgment. This is further complicated because hypocortisolism or other issues can increase the heart rate, sometimes due to increased adrenaline production.

- **Weight gain or loss** - gaining weight may suggest under-replacement of thyroid hormone. Weight loss can suggest having too high a dosage. Weight gain or loss is typically a slow process, but it is something to look out for, if there is any suspicion that thyroid dosage is not correct.

**Other specific tests that are worth doing:**

- **Listening to the heart for any abnormalities** - your doctor should do this is to ensure that the heart is not under strain from an incorrect thyroid dosage.

- **ECG (EKG)** - if there is any concern about the heart, an ECG should be done immediately. I would also suggest that anyone considering thyroid hormone treatment has an ECG done prior to treatment, for two reasons. Firstly, to ensure there are no previously undiagnosed heart abnormalities. Secondly, so that you have a baseline pre-treatment ECG to compare with later on. It is also a good idea to repeat the ECG once a stable, safe and effective thyroid dosage has been established, or at any time when there are concerns during treatment.

- **Serum Calcium Blood Test** - if thyroid hormone is too high, it can cause raised calcium in the blood. This occurs from bone loss, and must be detected and corrected. Symptoms include stomach upsets, constipation, frequent urination and impaired kidney function. So, it is very important to have a safe thyroid dosage. If calcium is high, check thyroid hormone dosage, using signs and symptoms.

- **Liver and Kidney Function Tests** - to ensure that these two organs are working effectively, these should be repeated occasionally, e.g. once the thyroid treatment is stable and then every few years. This is easy for your doctor to do.

- **Dexa Bone Density Scan** - should be carried out every few years to monitor any bone density changes. Having a Dexa scan every few years is important because this is the only way of comparing the current bone density with previous readings, to determine if any changes have occurred. If you can persuade your doctor to send you for a Dexa bone scan pre-treatment, this would be very good. You then know your bone density before you start treatment. If your doctor is concerned over your treatment and is worried about bone loss, the test can be repeated and a comparison made. Note: many doctors believe that a low TSH means a person is losing bone. In fact, more T3 does not cause bone loss. It simply speeds up all natural processes including bone turnover. Bone loss/gain depends largely on the hormones oestradiol, testosterone, and progesterone and to a lesser extent growth hormone. If these hormones are optimised, a good T3 level from any thyroid medication will increase bone formation and bone density more quickly.

- **Thyroid Lab Tests** - these also count as signs.

- **DIO1 and DIO2 genetic mutation tests** - these are very useful to do, even if you have to do them privately. Knowing that you have one or both mutations (and whether you have them from one or both parents), will inform you of the potential risk of conversion issues. Both mutations can reduce T4 to T3 conversion, lowering FT3 and raising rT3; thus increasing the chances of on-going hypothyroidism. Sometimes, the conversion problem only becomes apparent, as we get older; it is not clear within the field of genetics why this is. The **DIO1 mutation** may affect conversion by the thyroid, liver and kidneys. The **DIO2 mutation** may affect conversion by the brain, pituitary, central nervous system, thyroid, heart and peripheral tissues (skeletal muscle). **16% of thyroid patients are thought to have the DIO2 mutation**. The DIO2 mutation makes the D2 deiodinase enzyme faulty. D2 is significantly more effective in converting T4 to T3 than D1. Any reduced conversion capability, and especially through the **DIO2 mutation,** can also cause hypocortisolism, through the impact on the pituitary of lower T3 levels, i.e. due to HP dysfunction leading to lower ACTH. *If the DIO1 mutation is present, the liver is less effective in clearing rT3*.

Whatever company does the testing, it is important to ensure that they do report on the DIO1 and DIO2 mutations. So, ask them first before buying the test kit. *DIO1* is referred to as "rs11206244". The normal allele (no defect) is 'C'. The 'T' allele is the mutation; it reduces T4 to T3 conversion, and raises rT3 when active. *DIO2* is referred to as "rs225014". The normal/wild-type allele (no defect) is 'T'. The 'C' allele is the mutation; it reduces T4 to T3 conversion, and raises rT3 when active. Note - *Regenerus Labs* test for *DIO2* also (which is the most important of the two mutations, as the D2 deiodinase enzyme is far more efficient in converting T4 to T3 than the D1 deiodinase enzyme).

## LABORATORY TESTING

It can be extremely helpful to know which lab ran your tests for thyroid hormones, and other things like vitamins or minerals. Laboratory assays vary - a lot. Recording the lab used may prove useful later on. It is really only possible to compare one result with another, with any real authority, if they are from the same lab. *This is especially true with hormones like thyroid hormones or cortisol*. So, I also recommend making a note of this whenever you receive new lab test results. If you have copies of the results from the lab, please keep them, as they should have this information on them.

## THYROID HORMONE BRAND

Please keep a record with your symptoms and signs, regarding the brand of the thyroid medication being used. Brands vary in terms of potency and absorption. So, being able to access this information and know the brand and the dosage you were on when you recorded the symptoms and signs, and when you had the thyroid lab tests done can be very important.

## MORE SUBTLE POINTS ABOUT SYMPTOMS AND SIGNS

Over the years, I have learnt to listen to what my body is trying to tell me and I am now very in-tune with the messages it sends me. However, when I was trying to get well, I would use *signs and symptoms* to assess how well these changes in my thyroid medication were working.

As someone is getting close to their ideal thyroid hormone dosage, *symptoms* tend to be more subtle indicators of whether the dosage is right.

## TAKE THYROID MEDICATION AT THE SAME TIME EACH DAY

Whether you are using T4-Only, NDT, T4/T3 or T3-Only please do try to take your dose, or doses, at the same time(s) each day. This helps to make comparisons of symptoms and signs more practical. Setting alarms on a watch or on a cell-phone that you always have with you, can make this easier.

I used small containers, with reliably sealing lids, for any tablets that I needed when I was out of the house. I did not want to have to carry a lot of medication with me.

Having several of these are very useful, as you can leave one in a coat, another in a backpack or bag that you often have with you, and yet another in the car glove compartment. It is all too easy to go out and find that you have forgotten to bring any thyroid medication with you. Been there, done that and have the T-shirt!

## THYROID MEDICATION & SUB-LINGUAL USAGE

Sub-lingual use means allowing any thyroid medication to sit under the tongue, or next to the gum, and absorb there through the soft tissues of the mouth. It is intended to avoid any gut absorption issues.

However, I do not believe that this works at all. I talked to a thyroid researcher a few years ago about this and was told that the molecules of thyroid hormones (T4 and T3) are far too large to be absorbed that way.

Some thyroid patients believe that they have more success with their medication when taken this way. I believe that more saliva is produced when the tablet sits in the mouth for a while, but the thyroid medication still goes down the throat to the stomach. It just happens more slowly. If someone believes this provides a better result, they should probably continue doing so. However, I do not believe that it is sub-lingual absorption that is occurring.

My personal preference is to just chew up any thyroid medication before swallowing. I feel that this helps absorption.

Whatever method is taken to ingest the thyroid medication, it is important to do it consistently, as it may affect the tracking of symptoms and signs.

## TRACKING & RECORDING SYMPTOMS AND SIGNS

The approach will depend on which medication is being used. I will provide more suggestions in the individual chapters on each type of thyroid treatment. But in general, as someone moves from T4-Only to NDT or T4/T3 and then to T3-Only, they might need to move from 1-2 sets of measurement each day to 3-4 sets and then to 5-6 sets, when the thyroid dosage is being changed (titrated). Once stable on a dosage, regular measurement of symptoms and signs should not be required, unless something alters.

Here are some more points but they will still need to be refined later:

- Symptoms and signs are sometimes just called vitals or vital signs.
- Do not attempt to take readings before and after a CT3M dose, as this will disrupt sleep. CT3M works best with standard T3. It can be attempted with other medications like NDT, or with the T3 portion of T4/T3, but it is not as effective.
- Take a set of readings on waking/getting up, or within 30 minutes of getting up. Please try to record any significant changes in symptoms (improvements as well as any deterioration).
- Record readings 5-15 minutes before a daytime thyroid medication dose. This helps to see the *before dosing status*. This is particularly useful for medications that contain any T3 thyroid hormone.

- Record readings 2-3 hours after a daytime thyroid dose. For medications that contain T3 this will be invaluable. This is the *after dosing status.* It can show the affect on metabolism. With the before and after dosing status, it is usually possible to see how the T3 part of the medication is working.
- Record readings once in the evening e.g. 7 or 8pm.
- For T4-Only treatment, morning and afternoon readings may be sufficient.

**Here is an example of what a set of recordings for a day might look like:**

This example is for someone on T3-Only - so it is the most complicated of all.

\*\*\* START EXAMPLE \*\*\*

DATE: 8th March 2018

Date any T4/NDT Meds were Last Taken: 7 weeks.

TYPICAL GET UP TIME: 7:00 a.m. (This is important to know if CT3M is in use).

T3 Brand: Mercury Pharma T3

T3 Dosage:

20mcg T3 @ 07:00
10mcg T3 @ 11:00
10mcg T3 @ 14:00
10mcg T3 @ 17:00

SIGNS / VITALS:

| TIME | TEMP | HR | BP |
|------|------|----|------|
| 07:30 | 36.7 | 95 | 107/64 |
| 10:00 | 36.8 | 97 | 101/65 |
| 12:00 | 36.8 | 92 | 105/63 |
| 13:40 | 37.0 | 97 | 109/65 |
| 15:50 | 37.0 | 94 | 109/66 |
| 18:00 | 37.0 | 92 | 106/63 |

SYMPTOMS SUMMARY: Tired in the morning, with a headache. Did not sleep well previous night. Felt warm from 12 noon & a bit on edge in the afternoon. Had energy in the afternoon, and head felt clearer.

\*\*\* END EXAMPLE \*\*\*

The above is clear and organised and has only the essentials in it. This thyroid patient created a diary with time stamped (dated and timed) entries with this type of information, which made it easy for them to track progress after any thyroid medication change (in this case it was T3 medication).

Too much information, with many detailed descriptive comments, is almost as bad as too little, as it can be very difficult to understand it. Summarising the symptoms and signs collected into a few lines makes it easy to create a diary that the thyroid patient and their doctor can assess. When the information is summarised tidily, and in a short amount of space, any obvious patterns or results may be detected.

The type (brand) of thyroid medication being used, and the doses and timings, need to be recorded along with the signs (heart rate, body temperature and blood pressure, and any other laboratory test results). If there were lab test results, the name of the laboratory should also be recorded. As mentioned already, hormone assays vary by lab, so it is only possible to truly compare results from the same lab (unless the results are significantly different).

The typical time you get up should also be recorded. It is particularly important if you intend using CT3M. If you get up at 7:00 a.m. for 5 days of the week, and 9:00 a.m. at the weekend, record 7:00 a.m. for the typical get up time.

## HYPOCORTISOLISM / LOW NUTRIENTS CAN MASQUERADE AS HIGH / LOW THYROID HORMONE

In circumstances where cortisol or a nutrient is low, when your thyroid dosage is increased, you may feel more hypothyroid than before, e.g. body temperature may drop.

However, the opposite is also common. If one of these resources is very low, the increase in thyroid hormone dosage may also increase the symptoms and signs of excess thyroid hormones, including rapid heart rate or even raised blood pressure or body temperature. This may be caused in the case of hypocortisolism, by the adrenaline produced to compensate.

If body temperature, heart rate, blood pressure are normal, and no other adverse symptoms or signs are present, and if you feel well, you are extremely unlikely to be taking too much thyroid hormone. Thyroid lab tests can back that up, as long as they are interpreted correctly - see Chapter 14.

However, how you feel, and symptoms and signs, need to be centre-stage in any decision-making.

## CONSIDER SYMPTOMS, SIGNS & LAB TEST RESULTS TOGETHER

It is the viewing of all symptoms and all signs, including lab tests together that forms a picture. This is especially true after changes in thyroid medication or dosage.

## RESOURCES

Here is a list of further resources on this topic:

1. *Blog post summarising How to Track and Record Symptoms & Signs* - Paul Robinson. http://recoveringwitht3.com/blog/tracking-signs-and-symptoms-vitals
2. *Recovering with T3* - Paul Robinson. (It includes more information on symptoms and signs than I could include here).

# Chapter 14

# Thyroid Lab Test Results During Treatment

I have discussed all the thyroid blood tests and reference ranges in Chapter 8. They were relevant at that point because of trying to reach a diagnosis. We are now going to move into the treatment chapters. The way the thyroid blood test results are used during treatment is subtly different, and it varies with treatment type.

## THYROID LABORATORY TEST RESULTS VARY BY LAB

The ranges may vary slightly by laboratory. In some countries, or even in different labs within the same country, the units of measure may be different. So, you will need to use the ranges that your own lab provide when assessing the results.

It is also extremely important, if you want to compare results over time during treatment that you continue to use the same laboratory. For example, if you have FT3 tested at a new lab comparing this new FT3 level with past results from your previous lab with any degree of confidence, and comparing to previous and current symptoms will not be possible. When I say that each laboratory can vary, I do not mean by a small amount. The variations can be quite significant - see *reference 10* in Resources at the end of the chapter.

You also cannot compare your thyroid lab results to those of another group of people, or to another person. For example, those without a thyroid (due to surgery or advanced Hashimoto's), are an entirely different group, to those with a working thyroid gland. Even within a given group of people, individuals will vary. Imagine that someone with a thyroid gland had results X, Y and Z from the same laboratory as you use. They may be symptomless with these results. If you also have a thyroid, and during treatment your results are the same X, Y and Z, it does not mean that your symptoms will be resolved. You cannot compare the results of others to yours and draw conclusions.

You need to relate your own TSH, FT4, FT3 and rT3 thyroid lab results to each other during treatment. ***TSH, FT4 and FT3 are the minimal set of labs to be tracked at each blood draw***. If you can observe the way that the lab results change, and relate them to your symptoms and signs, using the guidelines in this book, you ought to be able to make fast progress. This should work well, as long as the laboratory and its assay method do not change.

Having said all the above, the rest of this chapter provides useful guidelines on how you can use the thyroid labs.

## FULL THYROID PANEL LABORATORY RANGES

I will begin with re-stating the laboratory tests and the reference ranges.

*Note: a thyroid panel must always be run first thing in the morning, prior to taking the first dose of the day of thyroid medication. So, do not take your thyroid medication on the morning of the blood tests (take it immediately after the blood draw). This includes any CT3M dose if you are using CT3M.*

In the UK the typical reference ranges for a full thyroid panel are:
- TSH:      (0.27–4.2) mIU/L
- FT4:      (12.0–22.0) pmol/L
- FT3:      (3.1–6.8) pmol/L
- RT3:      (10.0-24.0) ng/dL
- TPOAb: (< 34) IU/mL
- TgAb:     (< 40) IU/mL


In the USA the typical reference ranges for these are:
- TSH:      (0.5-4.70) µIU/mL
- FT4:      (0.8-1.8) ng/dL
- FT3:      (2.3-4.2) pg/mL or (80-180) ng/dL
- RT3:      (9.0-25.0) ng/mL
- TPOAb: (< 9.0) IU/mL
- TgAb:    (< 4 .0) IU/mL

## HOW TO USE THE THYROID LABS TEST RESULTS DURING TREATMENT

As I have said above, this will vary somewhat depending on the type of thyroid medication chosen.

Here are some common themes though:
- *TSH* - we know from research studies that for patients on T4-Only, symptom relief is usually associated with a TSH that tends to be near the bottom of the reference range, or sometimes below the low end (suppressed, near zero). However, this is not always the case. So, TSH alone is worthless, unless combined with the other more important thyroid labs and your symptoms. A very low or suppressed TSH is not a goal of treatment, and it may not be tolerated in some patients. However, it ought to be expected in many cases. This is true of all the different thyroid medications. Note: if someone was not on thyroid medication at all, a suppressed TSH might mean than they were hyperthyroid or even thyrotoxic, especially if FT4 and FT3 were raised and the person had symptoms. However, it is an entirely different situation for a

hypothyroid patient who is using thyroid medication to have a suppressed TSH - it does not imply too much thyroid medication is being given, or thyrotoxicosis is present. This is not the way many doctors view TSH currently. However, the research findings are fairly clear. See *references 1, 2, 3, 12 and 13* in Resources at the end of the chapter. *References 12 and 13* present articles written by eminent doctors in the UK, who are responsible, or influence, the treatment protocol for hypothyroidism. Both doctors acknowledge that TSH may be suppressed during treatment, and that this does not imply hyperthyroidism. They also make it clear that symptom relief is the goal of treatment. See *reference 14* also discusses this.

- *Free T4* - has the least correlation to symptom relief. However, we would expect it to rise in patients being treated with T4-Mostly therapies. FT4 is only useful in the context of how it alters with respect to the other thyroid hormone lab results during treatment. How symptoms change, and how the relationships of all the lab results change, is what is important. FT4 on its own, or FT4 with TSH, is of little use. Anecdotally, some thyroid patients have said that on T4-based therapies, they are optimal when FT4 is mid-range, or above. Equally, in a case of excellent conversion FT4 could be below mid-range. A specific FT4 level should not be a goal of treatment, as it is not correlated to symptom relief. See the *references 1 and 2* in Resources.

- *Free T3* - during treatment with thyroid hormone, the FT3 level relates more to symptoms than the other thyroid lab results. In most cases of successful treatment with any thyroid medication, patients appear to achieve optimal symptom relief with an FT3 level elevated into the upper half or even upper quartile of the FT3 reference range. Clearly, this cannot be achieved immediately, as the thyroid medication will need to be slowly and systematically increased. I would expect your FT3 to rise as your symptoms are being resolved. When symptoms are relieved, we should expect FT3 to be in the upper half of the range, or the top of the range during T4, NDT or T4/T3 based treatment. With T3-Only, expect FT3 to be near the top of the range, or even above the top (it will not imply thyrotoxicosis - more on this later). There will always be some exceptions of course - this is implicit in all my comments on lab tests. As ever, symptom relief is the most important aspect. See *reference 1* in Resources.

- *Reverse T3* - if progress is not going well, a conversion problem might be considered as a possibility. So, if FT3 is not increasing enough, or symptoms are not improving, testing FT3 and rT3 at the same time (same blood draw, so they are consistent in time), might be a good idea. A mid-range (or lower) FT3, and high rT3, would suggest there was a conversion problem, especially if someone is not improving after dosage increases. However, I do not believe there are any specific target levels for rT3, or an ideal ratio of FT3:rT3. You have to use common sense when interpreting the FT3 and rT3 levels together, perhaps seeing how they change during treatment, together with symptoms and signs. As mentioned earlier in the book, rT3 has been shown to be a T3-blocker. See the **references 4 and 5** in Resources.

- **TPOAb and TgAb** - these are often not tested again if Hashimoto's thyroiditis has been shown to be present. However, if you are working on strategies to lower these, retesting after 6 months or so might be useful. If TPOAb and TgAb were both negative, it might also be worth retesting in a couple of years, just to be certain that Hashi's has not developed. Generally though, we will not be concerned with the autoantibodies during treatment. Note: it is usually sensible to test only TPOAb, and if this is negative, to then test TgAb.

I need to continue to stress that it is symptoms, and key signs, like body temperature, heart rate and blood pressure that should be centre-stage throughout treatment. How these symptoms change, combined with the relationship of all the thyroid labs (including FT3) is what counts. *The focus should be patient-centric, not just lab-test-centric*.

### FT3 to FT4 ratio may offer some insights

Recent research proves that the ratio of FT3:FT4, for a given patient, is helpful to track during treatment. However, you must have results from the same lab (and the same assay technique within the lab), in order to compare the ratios. There are no absolute perfect numbers that apply to everyone. But for you, the way in which the ratio changes and relates to *your* symptoms is useful. You may feel wonderful with a particular FT3:FT4 ratio, whereas someone else may feel well with an entirely different ratio. FT3:FT4 ratio should increase as treatment progresses, and as symptoms improve. When all of your symptoms are resolved, you could choose to make a note of the ratio at that point. If any symptoms return in the future, you could re-check the ratio and compare with this to see if something has altered (as long as the same laboratory is being used).

Poor converters have a lower FT3:FT4 ratio, i.e. FT3 remains low in the range and FT4 remains high. This is also dosage dependent, due to the TSH relationship to conversion, i.e. the higher the dosage (especially if T4 dosage is higher), the lower the ratio is likely to be.

The FT3:FT4 ratio is particularly useful if you are going to require a *thyroidectomy*. It is known that after surgery the ratio is frequently lower due to the loss of the conversion capability of the thyroid gland; this can indicate the need for more T3 thyroid hormone. Having the before-surgery data, recorded along with symptoms, then comparing it with the after-surgery data, can be extremely useful.

Hashimoto's thyroiditis destroys thyroid tissue. It is slow and not as dramatic as surgery, but ultimately the effect can be the same. So, tracking the FT3:FT4 ratio can also be very insightful.

I explained in Chapter 4 that the loss of the thyroid gland through thyroidectomy or prolonged Hashimoto's results in the loss of the gland's deiodinases. The blood flowing through the gland can no longer have any FT4 content converted to FT3. It is not just the loss of the thyroid hormones produced by the thyroid gland that is a concern. Tracking the FT3:FT4 ratio, before and later, can be very helpful.

However, as stated, this is only useful if the tests are done within the same laboratory (and they have not changed the way the assay is being done). See **reference 9** in Resources.

### How often should thyroid lab tests be run?

This is dependent on the stage of treatment. During the early stages, thyroid labs are often run every 6-8 weeks. Later on, when someone is more stable, this happens far less frequently. It also depends on the type of treatment that is being used.

For more information on this, please refer to the treatment Chapters 15-19.

Please remember, thyroid labs should not be used to drive dosing decisions alone. Symptoms and signs should be centre stage.

## USE OF THE THYROID REFERENCE RANGES DURING TREATMENT

We know that the reference ranges are constructed from blood samples of people, who have TSH results that fit within the TSH reference range. There are two important points that I need to make.

*Firstly*, we know that many laboratories include the data from thyroid patients with in-range TSH levels. These thyroid patients are not screened to remove those who continue to have hypothyroid symptoms. Thyroid patients tend to have higher FT4 and lower FT3 than non-thyroid patients. This is because the T4-Only medication does not result in as much FT3 as a healthy person has from conversion of T4, plus there is a loss of T3 from the thyroid gland itself. It therefore takes more T4 medication to lower TSH into the reference range. The net-effect of this is that the bottom and the top of the reference ranges for FT4 and FT3 are influenced by the inclusion of the thyroid patient data. Some labs report a FT4 range of 0.8-2.2 ng/dL, when the non-thyroid patient range is 1.0 to 1.7 ng/dL. *As a result of this practice, you may be more likely to be considered healthy with lower biologically active thyroid levels than you really ought to have, i.e. higher inactive pro-hormone FT4 and lower biologically active FT3*. See **reference 11** and the **Reference Range Endocrinology** section within it.

*Secondly*, we also know, from recent research, that the current thyroid reference ranges (for TSH, FT4, FT3, rT3), are not the real reference ranges that each individual patient needs to have their hormones within in order to feel well. These **unique individual person reference ranges** are far narrower than the wide population ranges printed on current thyroid lab results. The **unique individual person ranges** are thought to be **less than half as wide** as the current thyroid lab reference/population ranges. See the last **references 6, 7 and 8** in Resources, for supporting research evidence of this.

Research has shown that once patients are on thyroid treatment, the required levels of thyroid hormones are not the same as in healthy people. Your unique individual reference ranges for the different thyroid hormones may have shifted from when you were healthy. This is another huge problem that exists within the current approach to treating thyroid patients. See the *reference 3* in Resources.

It is currently impossible to assess what the unique individual person ranges are, other than through the treatment of a thyroid patient. This is another huge issue, because in most instances, doctors are satisfied if the patient's thyroid labs sit within the population reference ranges - virtually anywhere within them!

Moreover, thyroid blood tests cannot measure the FT3, FT4 and rT3 levels within the cells. They only measure the blood portion and as such are an approximation to what might be present within the cells. Since conversion occurs within the cells we cannot know specific information about FT3, FT4 and rT3 inside the cells. So, treating symptoms and signs is key.

The bottom line is, there is not as much value to the thyroid lab reference ranges as is being assumed, and relied upon, by most doctors at the present time.

Simply having results that fit inside each lab test reference range is no guarantee of symptom relief. What is important, is finding a treatment regime that relieves your symptoms. *The response to treatment, and the changing relationships between TSH, FT4, FT3, and rT3 should be what guides dosing decisions.* Sticking mechanically to the existing reference ranges without using good clinical judgement is a desperately flawed approach. See also *reference 14* in Resources at the end of the chapter.

## FT3 REFERENCE RANGE FOR PATIENTS ON TREATMENTS WITH T3

I thought that I should share some thoughts on the FT3 reference range.

### How high should FT3 be in a blood test for a patient on T3-Only treatment?

Patients that require T3-Only, or T3-Mostly, treatment often come up against a big problem with doctors. Many doctors will not accept having a T3 dosage that puts FT3 blood test results over the top of the FT3 reference range. If this does happen, frequently the T3 medication is reduced or, in some cases, completely withdrawn!

The FT3 reference range used is derived from a population that includes treated thyroid patients. We know this incorrectly reduces the top of the FT3 reference range anyway.

The FT3 reference range being used *is exactly the same range as is used when treating people with T4-Only!* These people have T4 and T3 present in their bodies.

We know that many tissues in the body convert T4 to T3. The thyroid gland, the liver, kidneys, bones, muscles, the gut, the pituitary and brain all convert T4 to T3. This conversion occurs on an on-going basis over 24-hours. It occurs *within the cells* of these tissues! A good proportion of this converted T3 ends up being used within these cells, and never returns to the bloodstream at all. Some of the converted T3 does return into circulation, but it is thought that the bulk of the T3 is actually used within the cells where it was converted. However, researchers are still not sure of exactly how much is used within the cells and how much is returned to the bloodstream.

Consequently, the free T3 levels in a normal, healthy person, or someone on T4 medication, does not show how much FT3 the person has. Since FT3 in the cells cannot be measured, serum FT3 in a healthy individual is just an indicator of how much FT3 they really have, not the reality. The reality is that there is FT3 in the bloodstream, and there is FT3 created from FT4 that remains in the cells, but only the former can be measured. *If all the FT3 could be tested, the FT3 range would be far higher.*

To summarise, a normal person has on-going *sneaky* conversion of FT4 to FT3 occurring within the cells. This means that the FT3 reference range does not take account of the extra FT3 that they have gained from the FT4 (because a blood test can only test what is in the blood, and not what is inside the cells). So, the population reference range for FT3 only accounts for the circulating proportion of FT3 that actually exists for normal people. The real amount of FT3 is far higher.

In the case of patients using T3-Only treatment, or T3-Mostly treatment, they do not have on-going extra *sneaky* conversion of FT4 to FT3 going on within their cells. They have either little, or no FT4 at all. Of course, some of the circulating FT3 enters the cells and cannot be measured, but the on-going conversion from FT4 to FT3 does not happen!

Patients on T3 treatment are at a disadvantage in terms of the FT3 reference range because of this. *So, to restrict these patients on T3-Only treatment to the standard FT3 reference range is just silly! The reference range for someone with no FT4 should be higher to compensate for the loss of the converted FT3.*

Another way of saying all of this is that *someone who has much less than normal FT4 in their bloodstream has to have far higher FT3 levels to compensate.*

Note also: when someone is taking NDT, T4/T3 or T3-Only treatment, their FT3 levels will fluctuate markedly in relation to the time since the last dose. Making any sense of an FT3 test result in these cases is very hard anyway. For example, in the 8 hours after a T3 dose, FT3 is liable to be above the reference range in most people, but after 24 hours it may only be low in range. This is another reason to be wary of applying the FT3 reference range rigidly to people on treatment that includes T3.

My own experience with using T3 for over 20 years, and with my experience with thousands of thyroid patients, is that people on T3-Only therapy do well with reasonably high FT3 levels (often well above the top of the reference range).

Many thyroid patients who are on T3-Only are being *kept under-medicated and unwell* as a result of those doctors who attempt to apply the FT3 reference range rigidly. This is just wrong*!*

## What is the current state of understanding regarding all the above?

A few good doctors are sympathetic and understand that you cannot use the FT3 reference range to cap T3 dosage for those on T3-Only. However, they are not in the majority, and they are not setting the protocols for thyroid treatment. Many T3-Only patients that I speak to, are having a hard time from the doctors and specialists who are treating them. It is a very sad and upsetting situation. This is arising from a poor set of diagnosis and treatment protocols that make no allowances for a variety of thyroid medications and for recent research.

Tightly restricting treatment due to reference ranges that are not worth very much is an extremely poor way to go about things. People are being kept sick because of this practice!

## A NEW PARADIGM FOR THYROID HORMONE DIAGNOSIS & TREATMENT

I mentioned in Chapter 1 of this book that there is a need for a new paradigm of thyroid diagnosis and treatment. Most doctors are currently stuck in the TSH-T4 reference range paradigm from the 1970s. This is based on the assumption that almost all hypothyroidism is thyroid gland disease i.e. low thyroid hormones. They also believe that hypothyroidism can be treated simply by using T4 medication to normalise TSH and that a patient is adequately treated when TSH is in range. FT4, and if you are lucky, FT3 might also be somewhere in their reference ranges. When a doctor finally concludes that following the current paradigm is not resolving all the symptoms, they often declare that the patient has some other condition or disease. They never question the use of the current paradigm. This may not apply to all doctors who attempt to diagnose and treat hypothyroidism. However, it applies to an awful lot of them!

In this chapter and in others preceding it, I have begun to describe the new paradigm that must replace the current one. When you have read the entire book, you will have the recipe for what must form the core of the new paradigm for thyroid hormone diagnosis and treatment. This new paradigm needs to have more emphasis on the symptomatic response of the patient, with the proper use of lab testing in a supporting role. Moreover, the most suitable thyroid medication needs to be selected for each individual patient so that the best outcome is achieved.

## TRY TO AVOID PITFALLS & ROADBLOCKS

Most of this chapter challenges current medical practices. Many doctors are not patient centric, they are lab-test-centric. Many may not be happy to use the thyroid labs in the way I have suggested, because they were taught to apply them rigidly.

I expect that some of you who read this book and try to ask your doctors to work with them more in this way, may well find that you do not get the support that you need. However, as I keep saying, being forewarned is forearmed. You probably will not get what you need unless you ask for it, and are prepared to persuade your doctor in order to get it.

Being prepared for each medical appointment with all the main points that you need to mention will always help. Sometimes, writing a typed letter to your doctor well ahead of an appointment can be effective, as appointment slots appear to be getting shorter, and proper discussions are not always possible.

*Please try to get TSH, FT4 and FT3 tested as the minimal set each time you have a thyroid blood test.* Do continue to get hard copies of all your lab test results and, before each medical appointment, take the time to look through them and decide what they might mean. Continue to record which lab did your thyroid or cortisol tests. Your tracking of other symptoms and signs ought to help back up what you have to say to your doctor. It is *your* body and you need to try to ensure that it is looked after as well as possible.

Be on constant guard from TSH-centric, or thyroid-lab-result-centric doctors who think you are properly treated, when you are actually far from it. By reaching out to other patients, you may also have more of a chance of finding a good, empathetic doctor, should you need to find a new one. Sometimes changing your doctor can make a huge positive difference.

It can be a bit bumpy in the driver's seat at times. But armed with this book, you have a chance to take your car in the right direction!

## RESOURCES

Here is a list of research papers that back up many of the assertions made in this chapter:

1. *Symptomatic Relief is Related to Serum Free Triiodothyronine Concentrations during Follow-up in Levothyroxine-Treated Patients with Differentiated Thyroid Cancer* - Larisch, Midgley, Dietrich and Hoermann. See: https://www.thieme-connect.de/DOI/DOI?10.1055/s-0043-125064

   (This paper clearly proves that FT3 concentrations are the most important in clinical decision making, as they are most closely linked to residual hypothyroid symptoms in T4-Only treated patients. It also shows that in-range TSH is not sufficient for symptom relief.).

2. *Homeostatic equilibria between free thyroid hormones and pituitary thyrotropin are modulated by various influences including age, body mass index and treatment* - Hoermann R1, Midgley JE, Giacobino A, Eckl WA, Wahl HG, Dietrich JW, Larisch R. See: https://www.ncbi.nlm.nih.gov/pubmed/24953754

   (This is a great paper, although complex. It shows that it is the relationships of the thyroid hormones, and how they adjust during treatment, that counts. It also makes it crystal clear that TSH should only have a supporting role in the assessment process during treatment.)

3. *Recent Advances in Thyroid Hormone Regulation: Toward a New Paradigm for Optimal Diagnosis and Treatment* - Hoermann, Midgley, Larisch, Dietrich. See: https://www.frontiersin.org/articles/10.3389/fendo.2017.00364/full

   (This paper talks about the need for a new paradigm of thyroid treatment that accepts that the relationship between TSH and thyroid hormones are individual, dynamic and can adapt, i.e. the current practice of simply looking at numbers that do or do not fit in the population ranges is not sufficient).

4. *Qualitative and quantitative differences in the pathways of extrathyroidal triiodothyronine generation between euthyroid and hypothyroid rats* - J E Silva, M B Gordon, F R Crantz, J L Leonard, and P R Larsen. See: https://www.jci.org/articles/view/111313 (This paper shows that rT3 is a T3 blocker and not an inactive metabolite).

5. *The role of 3,3',5'-triiodothyronine in the regulation of type II iodothyronine 5'-deiodinase in the rat cerebral cortex* - Obregon MJ, Larsen PR, Silva JE. See:

https://www.ncbi.nlm.nih.gov/pubmed/3769868
(This paper also shows that rT3 is a T3 blocker and not an inactive metabolite).

6. *Narrow individual variations in serum T(4) and T(3) in normal subjects: a clue to the understanding of subclinical thyroid disease* - Stig Anderson. See: https://academic.oup.com/jcem/article/87/3/1068/2846746 (shows that individual person reference ranges are less than half as wide as the population lab test ranges).

7. *Reference range for thyrotropin. Post hoc assessment* - Larisch R, Giacobino A, Eckl W, Wahl HG, Midgely JE, Hoermann R. See: https://www.researchgate.net/publication/270645848_Reference_range_for_thyrotropin_Post_hoc_assessment

8. *Measurement of total rather than free thyroxine in pregnancy the diagnostic implications* - John E Midgley and Rudolf Hoermann. See: http://online.liebertpub.com/doi/abs/10.1089/thy.2012.0469?journalCode=thy

9. *Variation in the biochemical response to L-thyroxine therapy and relationship with peripheral thyroid hormone conversion efficiency* - Midgley, Larisch, Dietrich, and Hoermann. See: http://www.endocrineconnections.com/content/4/4/196.long

10. *Report of the IFCC Working Group for Standardisation of Thyroid Function Tests; Part 2; Free Thyroxine and Free Triodothyronine* - Beastall, Theinpoint, Toussaint and Uytfanghe See: https://www.researchgate.net/publication/43160144_Report_of_the_IFCC_Working_Group_for_Standardization_of_Thyroid_Function_Tests_Part_2_Free_Thyroxine_and_Free_Triiodothyronine

11. *Reference Range Endocrinology section* in Dr. Henry Lindner's submission to the Scottish Parliament. See: http://www.parliament.scot/S4_PublicPetitionsCommittee/General%20Documents/PE1463_C_Dr_Henry_Lindner_07.03.13.pdf

12. *Thyroid hormone replacement - a counterblast to guidelines* - Dr A.D. Toft. See: http://www.rcpe.ac.uk/sites/default/files/jrcpe_47_4_toft.pdf

13. *Consensus statement for good practice and audit measures in the management of hypothyroidism and hyperthyroidism* - M P J Vanderpump, J A 0 Ahlquist, J A Franklyn, R N Clayton, on behalf of a working group of the Research Unit of the Royal College of Physicians of London, the Endocrinology and Diabetes Committee of the Royal College of Physicians of London, and the Society for Endocrinology See: https://www.ncbi.nlm.nih.gov/pmc/articles/PMC2351923/pdf/bmj00557-0041.pdf

14. *Dr Henry Lindner Essay on thyroid treatment and use of lab tests* - http://www.hormonerestoration.com/Thyroid.html

# Chapter 15

## How to Use the Four Treatment Chapters

The next four chapters describe the main thyroid treatments. Each chapter is a standalone chapter, and does not require reading the other three in order to make sense.

- Chapter 16 covers treatment with T4-Only medication.
- Chapter 17 covers treatment with NDT medication.
- Chapter 18 covers treatment with T3-Only medication (but because this is a more difficult treatment, the **Recovering with T3** book is an essential read if you are planning to use T3-Only or T3-Mostly).
- Chapter 19 covers treatment with a mixture of T4 and T3 medication, i.e. T4/T3 treatment.

There are sections within the treatment chapters that are the same or very similar. I make no apology for this. If you read the chapters one after the other, you may well think that they are boring and repetitive. However, I did not write them to be read sequentially. I am expecting you to read the one that is currently most relevant to you.

Your doctor will have decided which treatment to begin with. I like to think that he has included you in the discussion about this, or at the very least, you have had a chance to ask some questions. There is little point reading about the other treatments immediately, as you will need to focus on the one you are about to use or are currently using.

However, if you do read them all at once, you will see the similarities of the chapters. I could have avoided this, but the result would have been more confusing. I decided it was better to have some duplication and make each chapter complete, and easier to read.

### A few words about slow-release T3

Slow-release T3 (SRT3) is a specially compounded version of T3, which releases slowly over time. However, it still peaks and troughs in the bloodstream, only not as quickly, or as high, as standard T3.

I have deliberately avoided writing a treatment chapter on SRT3, as I believe it is not suitable as a full treatment therapy for most people. I believe this for two reasons.

*Firstly*, when an SRT3 dose is taken, the T3 is released slowly over time. Getting it to peak fast enough to the right level, and yet not too high, is really difficult. Often, if the SRT3 is high enough to make someone feel well for a while, after a few hours, as the level builds up to too high a level, it can make the person feel unwell again

Conversely, if the SRT3 is low enough to avoid an unpleasant peak of T3, it can leave the person with hypothyroid symptoms for some of the time. Many thyroid patients have spoken to me over the years of their bad experiences with SRT3, when it has been prescribed as a full thyroid hormone replacement. Therefore, I am not giving it its own treatment chapter. If we could control the pattern of the release, i.e. programme it to meet our individual needs it would work well. However, we cannot. I hope some day that we can wear devices that release hormones in the ideal circadian pattern, tuned to our individual needs. We are just not there yet.

*Secondly*, in many countries SRT3 is very difficult to have prescribed. It often needs a specialised compounding pharmacy to make the SRT3 with the right dosage for the individual. Many doctors are simply not willing to prescribe it. Most, certainly in the UK, are not even aware of its existence.

However, SRT3 has a role in thyroid treatment. If someone is on T4-Only therapy, SRT3 can be added to this in small doses. I know of people who use T4 with the addition of one small morning dose of SRT3, or a morning and afternoon dose; they do very well on this.

If SRT3 was easily available, I might view it more positively. This day is not here yet.

In conclusion, I do not see SRT3 as a mainstream thyroid treatment. The other therapies provide full thyroid hormone replacement safely. So, I will not discuss SRT3 further.

## THE TYPICAL PROGRESSION OF TREATMENT

Almost everyone begins thyroid treatment with T4-Only (Levothyroxine or Synthroid). It may take many months before it is clear whether this treatment is likely to work or not. It should definitely be clear within one year whether it can provide full symptom relief (unless something else is confusing the issue).

If the T4-Only therapy is not successful, the two most obvious next treatments are either NDT or T4/T3. Your doctor is almost certainly going to have a preference. I personally, feel T4/T3 offers more flexibility in controlling how much of each hormone someone is getting.

Using either of these treatments will be a little harder than using T4-Only. However, they are easier to use than T3-Only. T3-Only is perfectly safe and very effective when used correctly. But T3-Only would require more effort on your part, and in the majority of cases it will not be required.

It may be six months to a year before you know if NDT or T4/T3 treatment is going to work well enough or not.

If there are still problems at that stage, you will have had symptoms for a long time. At that point I would buy the ***Recovering with T3*** book, read it, and urge your doctor to let you move on to T3-Only. When this is effective, there is always the option to attempt to add a little T4 back into the mix later on.

To summarise, the typical progression of treatments is usually likely to be:

1. T4-Only, then
2. T4/T3 or NDT, then
3. T3-Only

As mentioned many times earlier in the book, the biggest problem you may encounter may be your own doctor. Some of them are not open minded enough to switch medications. Some simply believe that all anyone needs is T4-Only. We know from experience, and from research, that the doctors that hold this view are totally wrong. However, you may have to contend with this. I have already discussed strategies to attempt to deal with this situation, should it arise.

Please also remember that T4 is not an active thyroid hormone. T3 is the biologically active thyroid hormone. If you have clear symptoms and signs of low thyroid effect, and your FT3 is not over the FT3 range on T4-Only therapy, you deserve a chance to try one of the other therapies that have added T3. You may need to make a big deal of this point with your doctor, who may actually not understand that T4 is an inactive thyroid hormone.

In conclusion, I have written the four treatment chapters in a way that you can just jump straight to whichever one you are using - they are entirely independent.

# Chapter 16

## T4 Treatment

In this chapter, I am going to refer to treatment with T4, with no added T3, as T4-Only, because it is simpler to write and easier to read. T4-Only is known as T4-monotherapy or LT4-monotherapy by doctors.

### WHAT EXACTLY IS T4?

T4 is the synthetic version of thyroxine, the biologically inactive thyroid pro-hormone. It can only do any truly useful task in the body if it converts efficiently to enough T3. As the dosage of T4 is raised, TSH is reduced, and the thyroid gland produces less T4 and T3. Your own thyroid produced its own T4 and T3, and a balance was achieved with TSH. Adding only T4, cannot achieve the same result. Thus, T4-Only thyroid medication is unlikely to provide the same level of biologically active T3 that your own thyroid used to do.

T4-Only is the first choice of the vast majority of doctors who treat hypothyroidism, and is often the only medication that they will prescribe.

The medication is also known by its generic name of Levothyroxine, or just Levo. There are well known brands too, e.g. Synthroid in the USA.

Tablets come in a variety of doses from 25-mcg, all the way up to 200-mcg, in increments of 25. They can all be split if needed.

### WHY CHOOSE THIS TREATMENT?

Although T4-Only treatment can sometimes work well, most experienced thyroid patients already know that it can leave many people with symptoms. In some cases, it can leave people with most of the symptoms that they began with.

T4-Only is probably the worst of all the available treatments, but it is often the only one offered.

On the upside, managing dosage is very straightforward, as it only needs to be taken once per day. It is also the cheapest of the treatments.

On the downside, it simply may not allow someone to recover. This will be compounded if the doctor involved is only looking at TSH to manage the treatment.

I would personally not recommend this form of treatment, but it is often very difficult to avoid it. The latter is the reason I have not included a special section in this chapter about how to swap to T4-Only from other thyroid treatments, as I consider the other treatments to be superior, because they provide some biologically active T3.

## TYPICAL FINAL DAILY DOSAGE OF T4-ONLY

After starting low and increasing slowly and carefully, a typical final replacement dose of T4-Only medication is frequently between 100 and 150 mcg. However, the dose can be as low as 75 mcg, or as high as 300 mcg in some patients. It is typical for people with higher body weight to require more T4 medication.

Older or more sedentary people may need less thyroid medication simply because their metabolism may be slightly slower. Moreover, people with heart issues are often kept on lower doses for safety reasons (although being hypothyroid is also a risk for those with heart problems).

## OTHER IMPORTANT BACKGROUND INFORMATION

T4 has a half-life. This is the time it takes for half of the amount in the blood to be eliminated. The half-life of T4 is 6-7 days for a healthy person, and 9-10 days for someone with hypothyroidism, whose metabolism is slower than a healthy person. The importance of this is that any T4-based therapy must allow time for any dosage change (increase or decrease) to stabilise. When you increase your dosage, you are adding more of the hormone each day, but the existing amount will reduce by half over the week. The bottom line is that it takes 8-12 weeks for total stability of the FT4 level in the bloodstream. However, after 4-6 weeks much of this stabilising has already occurred.

It is recommended that T4 medication be taken on an empty stomach. Ideally 30-60 minutes before a meal for completely optimal absorption. It is usually taken once per day, first thing in the morning. However, some people state that they do better when they take their daily dose at bedtime. There is some research evidence that lower TSH and higher FT4 levels are achieved when taking T4 at bedtime.

It is important to be aware, that as your FT4 level rises as the T4 dosage is increased, your TSH will usually fall. I explained in Chapter 7 that this would lower the conversion rate of FT4 to FT3. Consequently, it is possible that you will feel better after an increase of T4 dosage, only to find that some days later you feel just the same as you did before the raise. This is because there is an initial rise in FT3 due to more being converted from FT4. Then the thyroid itself produces less T4 and T3, and less FT3 is converted from FT4 due to the lowering of TSH. If this does happen to you, it may well occur after each dosage raise, until TSH is very low or close to suppression, i.e. below the lower end of the reference range - at that point the mechanism ceases to operate. This pattern may be seen in all T4-based therapies in some patients (although there are individuals who are better at converting than others, and are not as prone to this). However, for those with other T4 to T3 conversion issues this mechanism may prevent them from ever reaching a therapeutically effective dose of T3 medication.

In other patients, increases in T4 medication give little or no improvement due to poor conversion or other issues.

With T4-Only treatment the FT3 level tends to be lower than other therapies, particularly in patients without a thyroid gland, as they lack both the T3 production within the thyroid and the response to TSH in terms of conversion of FT4 to FT3 (within the thyroid itself). The latter point also applies to those who have suffered extensive thyroid tissue destruction through long-term Hashimoto's thyroiditis.

Selection of a good brand of T4-Only is important, because absorption varies across brands. Once on a brand that suits you, you should try to stick to that brand. Try not to let your pharmacist determine or change your brand.

T4 medication must be taken at least an hour or more before any calcium or iron supplement. If any iron or calcium supplement is taken, leave at least 4 hours clear before taking the T4 medication.

## START TRACKING SYMPTOMS AND SIGNS

I have already suggested that you begin to track symptoms and signs prior to taking any thyroid medication at all. This way, you will have a baseline, pre-treatment level. Comparisons can then be made to see how your treatment is progressing. I described how to do this in Chapter 13.

During T4 treatment, track symptoms and signs in the morning and afternoon on at least a few days each week.

Take more readings if things begin to get confusing or worrying. Making and keeping careful notes will be very useful indeed. You will be able to assess progress and watch out for problems. You will be able to summarise changes to your doctor and discuss the next steps.

## STARTING DOSE OF T4-ONLY

Doctors are likely to start adults on 25-50 mcg of T4 medication. There are some doctors who treat patients below the age of 60, who have no heart problems, with what they consider to be a full replacement dose based on the patient's weight alone. This latter approach has been carefully studied using 24-hour ECG monitoring.

Many doctors still use the ***starting low and raising the dosage slowly*** approach.

## WHEN TO INCREASE/DECREASE AND BY HOW MUCH?

Chapters 13 and 14 discuss all the most relevant information that can be used when assessing a T4-Only dosage change.

Typically changes are made in 25-mcg increments. However, based on symptoms and the full thyroid panel, a smaller or slightly larger change might be made. I use the word change because as someone approaches a dosage that resolves symptoms, it might be that the dosage gets a little too high after an increase and needs to be tapered down slightly.

Usually with T4-Only medication, dosage changes are made every 3-6 weeks, with 4 weeks being very typical. Most of the settling down of FT4 levels from the last increase will have occurred by then (not all, but the majority). If someone wanted to be utterly sure that the T4 level had stabilised, they would wait 8-12 weeks - this gap between dosage increases might be needed when you are very close to an optimal level. See the half-life discussion in 'Other Important Background Information', earlier in this chapter.

Waiting for longer periods between changes when the final dosage appears to be in reach might be an extremely sensible idea. I mentioned in Chapter 4, the genomic effects of T3 in the cell nuclei could take weeks or months to fully occur. This can be thought of as restructuring or reprogramming the genes. So, it sometimes takes patience in between increases to allow more time for this. Obviously, at the start of treatment the patient is often so short of thyroid hormone that it can be adjusted quite quickly. However, later on, more care and patience is required to allow the body enough time to adjust.

Note - even if TSH is fully suppressed, there will be some remaining, basal level of thyroid gland secretion of thyroid hormones. However, the effect of thyroid medication is that gradually, over time, this basal secretion will reduce. So, the thyroid medication level may need to be increased slightly as time goes on.

### WHEN SHOULD A FULL THYROID PANEL BE REPEATED?

Typically these are repeated every 8-12 weeks as the T4 medication is being adjusted.

Ideally, the whole panel of TSH, FT4, FT3 and rT3 should be done. *A minimal set of TSH, FT4 and FT3 ought to be run though.* However, many doctors only repeat TSH, which I have already said is inadequate. If things are not progressing well, you may begin to suspect conversion issues. In this case, getting FT3 and rT3 tested would be very helpful, even if you need to do this privately.

The full thyroid panel, *combined with symptoms*, should be used to drive dosage changes. This combination of information should also provide a skilled clinician with enough data to determine whether the T4-Only therapy is actually going to be successful in providing total symptom relief. It is very important to see FT3 as part of the thyroid lab test results. See Chapter 14 for interpretation of a full thyroid panel when under treatment.

*Thyroid blood tests must always be done first thing in the morning prior to the first dose of the day of thyroid medication.*

### SYMPTOMS AND SIGNS WHEN T4-ONLY DOSAGE IS IDEAL

Please refer back to Chapter 13 & 14 for more details - these are just the main highlights that are likely to be present when your T4-Only dosage is optimal:

- You should feel well and have relief from all hypothyroid symptoms.
- Body temperature should be normal for you - see Chapter 13.
- Heart rate should be normal for you.
- Blood pressure should be normal for you.
- Note: the important thing is how the labs and symptoms adjust during treatment with respect to each other. Every individual is unique in terms of where their levels will sit when symptoms are relieved. See Chapter 14 for more details.

- TSH could be near the bottom of the range or suppressed below it (but remember this is not always the case for some people, and it is not a goal of the treatment). Zero/suppressed TSH would not mean you are thyrotoxic on T4-Only, if your symptoms and signs are normal, and your FT3 is not over the top of the reference range (when you have taken the blood sample early in the morning prior to taking your T4 medication).
- FT4 could be mid-range or into the upper part of the range (this is not as important as FT3). In some cases, good T4 to T3 conversion may mean FT4 is below mid-range.
- FT3 is likely to be elevated into the top half of the range or near the very top. If FT3 is low in the reference range, this is a red flag if symptoms persist (even mid-range FT3 with many hypothyroid symptoms could suggest the treatment is not effective).
- RT3 should be low to mid-range and not high or over the top of the reference range.

## WHAT TO SUSPECT IF THERE ARE PROBLEMS?

It would be very unusual for no problems at all to appear during any thyroid hormone replacement. Some problems may not be thyroid hormone related. Symptoms and signs (Chapter 13) will often provide clues as to what the problem is.

Some of the basic things that can be wrong during treatment are:
- Not being on a high enough T4 dosage yet.
- Not absorbing the T4 medication properly, or not absorbing enough of it. Lab testing may also help to confirm this is happening. Low stomach acid or gut issues could have a bearing in this case, as can taking the thyroid hormone too close to calcium or iron.
- Not converting enough T4 to T3 (testing FT3 will show this, and testing FT3 and rT3 will show it further).
- Too much thyroid hormone. One would think that this would be easy to identify but sometimes, other issues cause the same symptoms. However, a combination of both symptoms and signs, including full thyroid labs, ought to be able to identify excess FT4 or FT3. Stepping back down in dosage for a while is always a possibility.
- Hypocortisolism, a low vitamin or mineral or some other issue that is interfering with treatment, and causing symptoms similar to the effects of either low or high thyroid hormone.
- Chapters 20, 21 and 22 provide further ideas, if all other issues have been totally ruled out.
- Being on the wrong type of thyroid hormone treatment for you! This very likely with T4-Only therapy.

Your doctor and you will have to work out which is the most likely and test that hypothesis. Further lab tests might have to be run, e.g. a cortisol saliva test for hypocortisolism. If cortisol is low, investigations might need to be done to find out why and correct it.

If the T4-Only treatment cannot be made to fully resolve symptoms, swapping to another thyroid treatment ought to be considered.

## WHAT TO DO WHEN YOU FEEL WELL

When you have full symptom relief, your task is not yet done. You need to make a very clear record of:

- All symptom improvements in as much detail as you can, so that you can compare if things change.
- All signs that you can measure now in good health - body temperature, heart rate, blood pressure.
- All signs related to test results now - vitamins, minerals, etc.
- Thyroid lab results now - TSH, FT4, FT3, and rT3.
- In particular, please pay close attention to how the relationships of the thyroid labs have changed from when you felt ill, to now when you feel well. If you can see these from the results, you will recognise what works for you as an individual. If things drift out of balance in the future, you will be able to recognise this far more easily.
- The FT3 to FT4 ratio.

Imagine a light switch, a separate dimmer switch and a light bulb. The switch and the dimmer control the brightness in the room. The brightness is going to be variable. So, getting the balance of thyroid hormones is much like this. Your personal dimmer switch has to be set just right. It is also going to be very individual. This is what I talked about earlier in the book, when I explained that your own personal thyroid levels for good health are unique to you, and that they may have altered from when you had no thyroid issues. See **reference 1 and 2** in Resources.

## TRY TO AVOID PITFALLS & ROADBLOCKS

There are more pitfalls & roadblocks possible within treatment itself than in any other aspect of recovering from hypothyroidism. They are too numerous to list.

If you have a supportive doctor and can work in partnership with them, you will be subject to far fewer pitfalls & roadblocks.

Tracking symptoms and signs at home will provide you with a lot of data that will show whether progress is being made or not. This will also reveal problems far sooner, and often more accurately, than a thyroid blood test panel.

Be prepared when you see your doctor at each appointment. This will help enormously.

Push to get a full thyroid panel when your blood tests are due to occur. Always get copies of the results, and record which lab did them. If you cannot get an rT3 test, look into doing FT3 and rT3 privately.

Please do not let your doctor drive your treatment using TSH alone, or even thyroid labs alone. Your symptoms and other signs are crucial in good clinical decision-making.

If you need a friend or relative to help you negotiate with your doctor, then teach them about hypothyroidism, loan them this book, and have them see your doctor with you at each appointment. Consider writing a simple letter prior to each appointment, so that you do not get stressed during the appointment and forget something important. Negotiate for what you need and why you need it within the letter.

Please also remember to make it clear to your doctor that T4 is not an active thyroid hormone. T3 is the biologically active thyroid hormone. If your T4-Only treatment is not working well, a trial of one of the other therapies may well be needed.

Worst case, if your doctor is dogmatic, does not take your needs on board, or is committed to using thyroid labs to manage your treatment, work hard to find a better one.

If you want to get well as quickly as possible, you will need to get involved and gain some control of your health.

## RESOURCES

Here is the research paper that discusses how an individual patient will have a unique set of relationships between the thyroid hormones and TSH:

1. *Recent Advances in Thyroid Hormone Regulation: Toward a New Paradigm for Optimal Diagnosis and Treatment* - Hoermann, Midgley, Larisch, Dietrich. See: https://www.frontiersin.org/articles/10.3389/fendo.2017.00364/full
   (This paper talks about the need for a new paradigm of thyroid treatment that accepts that the relationship between TSH and thyroid hormones are individual, dynamic and can adapt, i.e. the current practice of simply looking at numbers that do, or do not, fit in the population ranges, is resulting in poor patient care).

2. *Narrow individual variations in serum T(4) and T(3) in normal subjects a clue to the understanding of subclinical thyroid disease* - Stig Anderson. See: https://academic.oup.com/jcem/article/87/3/1068/2846746

# Chapter 17

## NDT Treatment

NDT treatment stands for natural desiccated thyroid treatment.

### WHAT EXACTLY IS NDT?

The first successful treatment of hypothyroidism occurred in 1891. A patient was cured of severe hypothyroidism with injections of animal thyroid gland extract. Later on, porcine (pig) thyroid extracts were used and mass-produced. Natural desiccated thyroid (NDT) remained the main treatment for hypothyroidism until the 1960s.

In the late 1960s, encouraged by the company that makes Synthroid (synthetic T4), the big switch over began to happen. NDT went out of favour and T4 medication took over, as pharmaceutical company representatives persuaded doctors to switch to T4 for thyroid treatment.

NDT tablets are usually measured in grains e.g. 1 grain, 2 grains, 3 grains etc. They can also be split and given in half grains. 1 grain of NDT is sometimes measured as 60 mg of NDT, e.g. 30 mg of NDT would be 1/2 a grain.

In 1 grain of NDT there is typically 38 mcg of T4 and 9 mcg of T3. This is about a 4:1 ratio, which is unlikely to be the same as the human thyroid gland produces. Whatever our real ratio of T4:T3 from a healthy human thyroid is, we know that it is variable and controlled. See Chapter 4 for more information on our thyroid gland and its hormones.

Note: there may be slight differences in the above numbers in some brands of NDT. It would be best to check with other thyroid patients regarding any brand of NDT that you are considering using, or that your doctor is prescribing.

The T4 and T3 within NDT are bound to the thyroglobulin protein and are not free, as in synthetic T4 or T3. They only become free hormones after they are digested in the small intestine. However, doctors still state there are high peak levels of FT3 following NDT doses and lower trough levels; so, the absorption is not dissimilar to synthetics T4 and T3.

NDT also contains T2, T1 and calcitonin, which you do not get with T4 medication. I explained in Chapter 4 that those on T3-only, or any T4/T3 medication, would produce all the T2 and T1 that they need, through the deiodination of T3. Calcitonin is also thought to have little importance.

### WHY CHOOSE THIS TREATMENT?

NDT is still thought by many to be the most effective thyroid treatment for those thyroid patients that convert FT4 into FT3 reasonably well. Porcine thyroid hormones are identical to human thyroid hormones, so it is more natural than T4-Only, and more effective because it contains T3 in addition to T4There is a lot of anecdotal evidence that suggests patients tolerate NDT and do far better on it than other thyroid treatments. One of the most powerful arguments is that because NDT contains T3, it is more physiological and can help those with T4 to T3 conversion problems.

The other point to note is that, having some T3 in the mix, provides more stability in the TSH and thyroid hormone system. The level of TSH affects the conversion rate of T4 to T3, as I have described several times now. T3 is naturally more suppressive of TSH than T4. What we do not want is TSH to be oscillating high and then low, as thyroid hormone levels rise after a T4-Only dose, then fall again over the day. The addition of T3 brings a much-needed stability to the entire system. See *reference 5* in Resources at the end of this chapter (only the abstract is available as I write this, as it is a 2018 published study).

## TYPICAL FINAL DAILY DOSAGE OF NDT

After starting low and increasing slowly and carefully, a typical final replacement dose of NDT medication for adults is frequently between 2 and 5 grains, with most needing 3-3.5 grains. It is typical for people with a higher body weight to need more thyroid medication.

As with T4-Only, older or more sedentary people may need less thyroid medication simply because their metabolism may be slightly slower. Moreover, people with heart issues are often kept on lower doses for safety (but being hypothyroid is a risk for those with heart problems).

## OTHER IMPORTANT BACKGROUND INFORMATION

The T4 content of the NDT has a half-life. This is the time it takes for half of the amount of the T4 in the blood to be eliminated. The half-life of T4 is 6-7 days for a healthy person, and 9-10 days for someone with hypothyroidism, whose metabolism is slower than a healthy person. The importance of this is that any T4-based therapy must allow time for any dosage change (increase or decrease) to stabilise. When you increase your dosage, you are adding more of the hormone each day, but the existing amount will reduce by half over the week. The bottom line is that it takes 8-12 weeks for total stability of the FT4 level in the bloodstream. However, after 4-6 weeks much of this stabilising has already occurred.

NDT can be taken on an empty stomach or not. However, if you have any concerns about absorption, then taking it on an empty stomach 30-60 minutes before food would be safer.

NDT is usually taken twice, or sometimes 3 times per day, to spread out the doses of T3 that are within the NDT. It is not usually taken all in one dose in the morning, because the T3 content would be likely to be too potent and cause problems, e.g. faster heart rate, raised blood pressure, anxiety and jitteriness etc. However, some people argue that, because the hormones in NDT are bound to protein (unlike synthetic T4 and T3), it is acceptable to take it once a day. It is important to be aware that the hormones become free after they are digested, and this is likely to result in a large rise in T3 early in the day. This in itself would not be physiological, but it might be tolerated by some patients.

It is important to be aware that as your FT4 level rises in response to increases in NDT medication, TSH will usually fall. Consequently, you may feel better after an increase of NDT, only to find that some days later you feel just the same as you did before the raise. This can occur for a while on low doses of NDT. However, as the medication level rises after dosage increases, the increasing T3 that comes from the NDT each day should begin to stop this effect.

NDT medication must be taken at least an hour or more before any calcium or iron supplement. If any iron or calcium supplement is taken, leave at least 4 hours clear before taking the NDT medication.

## START TRACKING SYMPTOMS AND SIGNS

I have suggested that you begin to track symptoms and signs prior to taking any thyroid medication at all. This way, you will have a baseline, pre-treatment level. Comparisons can then be made to see how treatment is progressing. I described how to do this in Chapter 13.

During NDT treatment, because you are now ingesting T3 medication, I would advise tracking symptoms and signs. You should take readings in the morning when you wake/get up (before your NDT dose), then 2-3 hours later, then again before your afternoon NDT dose and 2-3 hours later, then perhaps in the evening. I recommend doing this on 2-4 days of the week, not necessarily every day.

Take more readings if things begin to get confusing or worrying. Making careful notes and keeping them will be very useful indeed. You will be able to assess progress and watch out for problems. You will be able to summarise changes to your doctor and discuss the next steps.

## STARTING DOSE OF NDT

There is some debate about the best starting dosage. Dr. Mark Starr is a physician who specialises in thyroid issues. He also wrote the book in **reference 3** in Resources. Dr. Starr recommends that adults start with between 0.25 and 0.5 grains of NDT medication. Janie Bowthorpe, who wrote the book in **reference 4**, recommends 1 grain as a good starting level. If cortisol has been tested, and is at a good level, starting with 1 grain is probably fine. However, if you have not tested cortisol, please start lower, to avoid problems if cortisol was actually low.

Dr. Starr's argument is that many adults these days have toxicity issues and need time to get accustomed to the increased level of T3, which results from the NDT. However, I do not know if he uses multi-dosing, which is recommended. I see no problems with starting low, as long as you are prepared to increase quickly if you remain, or become more, hypothyroid.

When starting with 0.5 or 1 grain per day of NDT, this need only be split into 2 divided doses. It is suggested that 2/3 of a grain is taken in the morning, when you get up, and the other 1/3 in the early to mid afternoon. If for any reason this is not tolerated well, it could be reduced quite quickly by halving each of these doses.

The 2/3 and 1/3 proportions, when 2 divided doses are being used, fits well with the natural pattern of FT3 that is higher in the morning and lowers during the day.

## WHEN TO INCREASE/DECREASE, BY HOW MUCH AND TO WHICH DOSE?

Typically, thyroid patients on NDT increase by 1/2 grain every 2-3 weeks during the start of treatment. An increase of 1/2 grain is equivalent to 19 mcg of T4 and 4.5 mcg of T3. This could be varied slightly depending on symptoms and signs (see Chapter 13).

When someone reaches 2 grains per day, the time between dosage increases should be longer. This is because the body needs time to adjust to the increases of T3. It is also because some patients may not need much more than this. Remember, the T4 content of NDT has a half-life of about a week, so it needs 4-6 weeks to mostly stabilise (8-12 weeks to fully stabilise).

Consequently, once a patient has reached 2 grains per day, adding another 1/2 grain every 4-6 weeks is usually recommended.

However, based on symptoms, and the full thyroid panel, a smaller or slightly larger change might be made. I use the word change because, as someone approaches a dosage that is resolving symptoms, it might get a little too high and need to be tapered down slightly.

As the dosage of NDT appears to get closer to therapeutic levels, the time between increases can get extended. Allowing sufficient time for the T4 content to build up and stabilise is essential at this stage (if another increase is done too soon, you could over-shoot the ideal dosage). As with T4-Only, this is likely to be 8-12 weeks, but it could be longer when most of your symptoms have been eliminated.

I mentioned in Chapter 4, the genomic effects of T3 in the cell nuclei could take weeks or months to fully occur. This can be thought of as restructuring or reprogramming the genes. So, it sometimes takes patience in between increases, especially when the dosage is closer to a therapeutic level. The body needs the time to adjust. Note - the effect of thyroid medication is that gradually, any basal thyroid secretion will reduce. So, the thyroid medication level may need to be increased slightly as time goes on.

## MULTI-DOSING

As already mentioned, NDT is usually multi-dosed. 2 doses per day are fairly standard. Once the total daily dose of NDT has exceeded 3 grains, it is possible for this to be switched to 3 doses per day. The decision should be made on how well the NDT is being tolerated. Some patients are able to tolerate a single dose of NDT when they wake up.

If 3 doses are used, dosing might be done first thing in the morning, late morning or just after lunch and mid to late afternoon. If this were done, ideally 2/3 of the daily dose would be provided in the first 2 doses and the other 1/3 in the last dose. Symptoms and signs can help make this decision. Every individual is different, so these are just guidelines.

## WHEN SHOULD A FULL THYROID PANEL BE REPEATED?

Typically these are repeated every 8-12 weeks, much like the T4-ONLY medication.

A full panel including TSH, FT4, FT3 and rT3 should be done. ***A minimal set of TSH, FT4 and FT3 ought to be run though.*** However, many doctors only repeat TSH. This is a huge issue as discussed already. If things are not progressing well you may begin to suspect conversion issues. In this case, getting FT3 and rT3 tested would be very helpful, even if you need to do this privately.

The full thyroid panel, **combined with symptoms**, should be what is used to drive dosage changes. Please ensure FT3 is tested as part of the thyroid panel. See Chapter 14 for interpretation of a full thyroid panel when under treatment.

*Thyroid blood tests must always be done first thing in the morning prior to the first dose of the day of thyroid medication. This includes any CT3M dose if you are using CT3M.*

## DOSING - IF SWAPPING FROM OTHER THYROID MEDICATION

The usual recommendation, if swapping from T4-Only to NDT, is to just swap over completely within 24 hours, i.e. finish taking the T4 on one day and start the NDT on the very next day.

The starting dose regime for the NDT is exactly the same as described above, i.e. you start low (do not try and guess the equivalent dose of NDT to the T4-Only dose you were previously taking). The reason for this is safety. The biologically active T3 within the NDT can be very stimulatory, and takes time to get used to. So, starting low is important. Having the active T3 present in the NDT can also help to make the built-up T4 in your body convert better. Hence it is best to be very careful.

However, if hypothyroid symptoms begin to return quickly, less time could be allowed between some of the first few dosage increases.

## SYMPTOMS AND SIGNS WHEN NDT DOSAGE IS IDEAL

Please refer back to Chapter 13 & 14 for more details - these are just the main highlights that are likely to be present when your NDT dosage is optimal:

- You should feel well and have relief from all hypothyroid symptoms.
- Your body temperature should be normal for you - see Chapter 13.
- Heart rate should be normal for you.
- Blood pressure should be normal for you.
- Note: the important thing is how the labs and symptoms adjust during treatment with respect to each other. Every individual is unique in terms of where their levels will sit when symptoms are relieved. See Chapter 14 for more details.
- TSH could be near the bottom of the range or suppressed below it (but remember this is not always the case for some people, and it is not a goal of the treatment).
- FT4 is likely to be mid-range but could be low in the range or slightly above mid-range when tested before the first morning dose of NDT. In some cases, good T4 to T3 conversion may mean FT4 is below mid-range. There is no need to try to get FT4 high in the range (where it is more likely to create too much rT3).
- FT3 is very likely to be elevated into the top half of the range or near the very top.
- RT3 should be low to mid-range and not high or over the top of the reference range.

### THE CIRCADIAN T3 METHOD (CT3M) CAN BE USED WITH NDT

In the case where there is hypocortisolism, the first dose of NDT could be used to implement the CT3M protocol. This sometimes works, even with NDT medication, although T3 is usually more effective. Find out a little more about CT3M in Chapter 18 (T3-Only Treatment), and in *Recovering with T3* and *The CT3M Handbook*.

### WHAT TO SUSPECT IF THERE ARE PROBLEMS?

It would be very unusual for no problems at all to appear during any thyroid hormone replacement. Some problems may not be thyroid hormone related. Symptoms and signs (Chapter 13,) will often provide clues as to what the problem is.

Some of the basic things that can be wrong during treatment are:

- Not being on a high enough NDT dosage yet - being overly slow at increasing it. Due to the effect of lowering TSH affecting conversion, this can cause someone to stay hypothyroid even longer, or get even more so. Tracking symptoms and signs will help to avoid this.

- Not absorbing the NDT properly, or not absorbing enough of it. Begin to suspect this if there is no symptomatic response during the day after NDT doses, and especially if you have raised a dose. Lab testing may also help to confirm this is happening. Low stomach acid or gut issues could have a bearing in this case, as can taking the thyroid hormone too close to calcium or iron.

- Not converting enough T4 to T3 (testing FT3 will show this, and testing FT3 and rT3 will show it further). This could turn into a big issue if the cause of the poor conversion cannot be found and corrected.

- Too much NDT hormone. Usually caused by trying to get to a therapeutic dosage too quickly. One would think that this would be easy to identify, but sometimes, other issues cause the same symptoms. However, a combination of both symptoms and signs, including full thyroid labs, ought to be able to identify excess NDT. Stepping back down in dosage for a while is always a possibility.

- Trying to use only one dose per day of NDT can also cause big issues. That dose can have far too much T3 content. Furthermore, this is not a physiological replacement method, as the body would produce some extra T3 over the day (from the thyroid gland and through conversion from T4).

- Not tracking symptoms and signs, and only going on thyroid labs to guide dosage changes.

- Hypocortisolism, a low vitamin or mineral or some other issue that is interfering with treatment, and causing symptoms similar to the effects of either low or high thyroid hormone. Consequently, some or all of the pre-treatment tests could be run again.

- Chapters 20, 21 and 22 provide further ideas, if all other issues have been totally ruled out.

- Sometimes, with all the will in the world, NDT may not be right for an individual.

Your doctor and you will have to work out which is the most likely and test that hypothesis. Further lab tests might have to be run, e.g. a cortisol saliva test for hypocortisolism. If cortisol is low, investigations might need to be done to find out why and correct it.

If the NDT treatment cannot be made to fully resolve symptoms, swapping to another thyroid treatment ought to be considered.

## WHAT TO DO WHEN YOU FEEL WELL

When you have full symptom relief, your task is not yet done. You need to make a very clear record of:

- All symptom improvements in as much detail as you can, so that you can compare if things change.
- All signs that you can measure now in good health - body temperature, heart rate, blood pressure.
- All signs related to test results now - vitamins, minerals, etc.
- Thyroid lab results now - TSH, FT4, FT3, and rT3.
- In particular, please pay close attention to how the relationships of the thyroid labs have changed from when you felt ill, to now when you feel well. If you can see these from the results, you will recognise what works for you as an individual. If things drift out of balance in the future, you will be able to recognise this far more easily.
- The FT3 to FT4 ratio.

The balance of your thyroid lab results is going to be unique to you, and they may vary over time. This is what I talked about earlier in the book, when I explained that your own personal thyroid levels for good health are unique to you, and that they may have altered from when you had no thyroid issues. See *references 6 and 7* in Resources.

## TRY TO AVOID PITFALLS & ROADBLOCKS

There are more pitfalls & roadblocks possible within treatment itself than in any other aspect of recovering from hypothyroidism. They are too numerous to list.

If you have a supportive doctor and can work in partnership with them, you will be subject to far fewer pitfalls & roadblocks.

Tracking symptoms and signs at home will provide you with a lot of data that will show whether progress is being made or not. This will also reveal problems far sooner, and often more accurately, than a thyroid blood test panel.

Be prepared when you see your doctor at each appointment. This will help enormously.

Push to get a full thyroid panel when your blood tests are due to occur. Always get copies of the results, and record which lab did them. If you cannot get an rT3 test then look into doing FT3 and rT3 privately.

Please do not let your doctor drive your treatment using TSH alone, or even thyroid labs alone. Your symptoms and other signs are crucial in good clinical decision-making.

If you need a friend or relative to help you negotiate with your doctor, then teach them about hypothyroidism, loan them this book, and have them see your doctor with you at each appointment. Consider writing a simple letter prior to each appointment so that you do not get stressed during the appointment and forget something important. Negotiate for what you need and why you need it within the letter.

If NDT is not resolving your thyroid issues, and no other problem can be found, trying one of the other therapies will be needed. Use the information in the other treatment chapters to explain the benefits of these to your doctor. They may be persuadable.

Worst case, if your doctor is dogmatic, does not take your needs on board, or is using thyroid labs only, work hard to find a better one.

If you want to get well as quickly as possible, you may well need to get involved and gain some control of your health.

## RESOURCES

Here is a list of further reading for those who wish to gather more background on some of the topics in this chapter:

1. ***Recovering with T3*** - Paul Robinson. (See information on the Circadian T3 Method - CT3M).

2. ***The CT3M Handbook*** - Paul Robinson. (More information on CT3M).

3. ***Hypothyroidism Type 2*** - Mark Starr, M.D. (Chapter 9 Treatment Guideline - My Recommendations by Mark Starr).

4. ***Stop the Thyroid Madness*** - Janie A Bowthorpe, M.Ed. (Discusses NDT).

5. ***Mathematical modelling of the pituitary-thyroid feedback loop: role of a TSH-T3-shunt and sensitivity analysis*** - Berberich, Dietrich, Hoermann and Muller.
   See: https://www.frontiersin.org/articles/10.3389/fendo.2018.00091/abstract
   (The full article is not available yet, but this paper shows how T3 helps to stabilise the TSH-thyroid hormone system).

6. ***Narrow individual variations in serum T(4) and T(3) in normal subjects a clue to the understanding of subclinical thyroid disease*** - Stig Anderson.
   See: https://academic.oup.com/jcem/article/87/3/1068/2846746

7. ***Recent Advances in Thyroid Hormone Regulation: Toward a New Paradigm for Optimal Diagnosis and Treatment*** - Hoermann, Midgley, Larisch, Dietrich. See: https://www.frontiersin.org/articles/10.3389/fendo.2017.00364/full
   (This paper talks about the need for a new paradigm of thyroid treatment that accepts that the relationship between TSH and thyroid hormones are individual, dynamic and can adapt, i.e. the current practice of simply looking at numbers that do, or do not, fit in the population ranges, is resulting in poor patient care).

# Chapter 18

## T3 Treatment

In this chapter, I am going to refer to treatment with T3, with no added T4, as T3-Only because it is simpler to write and easier to read. T3-Only is known as T3-monotherapy or LT3-monotherapy by doctors.

### WHAT EXACTLY IS T3?

T3 is the synthetic version of triiodothyronine, the biologically active thyroid hormone. In my other books, I have also referred to this as Standard-T3 or Pure-T3, as opposed to Slow-Release-T3 (SRT3). I am not going to discuss SRT3, as it is more difficult to get prescribed and harder to use as a full thyroid hormone replacement. T3-Only is fast acting and needs to be multi-dosed over the day, much like NDT needs to be. Because each T3-Only dose can be tailored in terms of dose size and timing, it can be used to create a safe and effective overall dosage that never causes tissue over-stimulation.

The generic name for the medication is Liothyronine Sodium, and often, just Liothyronine. There are numerous brands including: Cytomel, Cynomel, Tiromel and Thybon. Some brands are thought to be slightly stronger than others.

Depending on the generic or brand, T3-Only comes in limited sized tablets, typically only 20-mcg or 25-mcg. Frequently, thyroid patients have to halve or quarter these when trying to keep any dose increases at a safe level.

It is very important to be aware that T3 is far more potent than T4 - at least 10 times more potent when researchers have studied T3 and T4. T3 also binds far more easily to the thyroid receptors; hence the effective potency of T3 is far higher than a factor of 10 over T4. However, in a good converter of T4, some T3 is produced, which tends to make this fact less obvious.

T3 also converts within the body to T2 and T1, so there will be sufficient amounts of both of these for those people using T3-Only.

### WHY CHOOSE THIS TREATMENT?

T3-Only treatment is usually the last one to be selected - I agree with this choice, as it is more difficult to manage. *I often refer to T3-Only as the treatment of last resort.* It is only really considered, if one or more of the other treatments fail to work well enough. However, most doctors and endocrinologists will not prescribe it. They believe it is unnecessary, because they think all patients always get enough T3 from conversion of T4. Thus most doctors think that T4-Only is sufficient. This is clearly wrong.

T3-Only does not need to convert to anything to increase metabolism within our cells. It is already in the ***biologically active form***. So, for someone with a conversion issue, it can completely get around this problem. As mentioned in Chapter 4, the Watts Study found that a significant proportion of thyroid patients have a genetic defect of the DIO2 gene that significantly hampers T4 to T3 conversion. This is just one possible cause of faulty conversion.

Incidentally, I have recently had DIO1 and DIO2 tested myself. Apparently, I have both mutations. I also inherited each from both my parents. The mutations ensure that I produce faulty D1 and D2 deiodinase enzymes, leading to T4 to T3 conversion issues. This, together with the loss of the conversion by my thyroid gland (because it was destroyed by Hashimoto's thyroiditis), goes some way to explain my own situation. Note: the pituitary gland, which produces ACTH, uses the D2 enzyme to convert 80% of the T4 within its cells to T3. It needs high T3 levels to function. Because of this, it is easy to see why I might also have had hypocortisolism. The liver uses D1 to clear rT3; so, I would also have been prone to high rT3.

Some patients never get symptom relief without using T3-Only. I have worked with thousands of them and I know this to be a fact. The proportion of patients who need T3-Only, compared to those who are able to get well with one of the other thyroid therapies, is very small. However, for these people, T3-Only can help them to fully recover from hypothyroidism. I am one of those who needs T3-Only to be healthy.

I have been on T3-Only for over 20 years. It works very well for me. I have tried to use T4, but even a small amount makes me very ill. This book will not go into all the possible reasons for this, as it is intended to be a practical manual.

T3 is potent and has to be ***multi-dosed*** for safety, and to provide a more physiological (natural) rhythm of T3 level over the day. Even then, there will be peaks and troughs due to the way the individual doses work. It is therefore harder to dose than the other treatments, and as such, it should be the last treatment that you and your doctor consider.

Most doctors are reluctant to prescribe T3, so it may be difficult to find a competent, sympathetic doctor who will. Then, learning to use it safely is paramount.

My ***Recovering with T3*** book provides a ***safe and effective protocol for using T3***. For those considering T3-Only, it remains the go-to book on the subject. In the interest of using T3 safely, I recommend that you read it, and do not rely on this book alone. It was not possible to distil a large book like ***Recovering with T3*** into a small chapter like this.

## TYPICAL FINAL DAILY DOSAGE OF T3-ONLY

After starting low, and increasing slowly and carefully, a typical final replacement dose of T3-Only medication for adults is frequently between 40 and 80 mcg. However, some patients need less and others need more. I personally know several people who require 150-200 mcgs of T3 per day, and they have not got any hyperthyroid (thyrotoxic) symptoms at all. However, this type of dosage is not common.

It is typical for people with higher body weight to require more thyroid medication. Older or more sedentary people may need less simply because their metabolism may be slightly slower. Moreover, people with heart issues are often kept on lower doses for safety reasons (although being hypothyroid is also a risk for those with heart problems).

The total daily dosage of T3 is usually taken in 3 divided doses. However, some patients use only 2 divided doses, and some need 4 or more divided doses. Very rarely, it is all taken in one dose, but I do not recommend this, as it is not a physiological way to introduce T3 into the body.

## THYROID LABS ARE OF LIMITED USE IN MANAGING T3-ONLY DOSING

A full thyroid panel is going to be of limited use to you and your doctor regarding what dosage changes to make, or whether you are on the correct amount of T3. This may disturb some doctors who like to believe that they can arrive at the ideal dosage just using TSH, or even FT3. Some other doctors may also be perturbed to see your FT4 level plummeting towards zero. T3-Only is a very different therapy; the guidelines for using the other thyroid hormones cannot be applied to this medication.

In the majority of cases of using T3-Only, all the other treatments have already failed abysmally. There is clearly something very different about the group of people who find that they need to use T3-Only.

For this group, symptom relief usually only comes with a daily dosage of T3 in the 40-80 mcg range. These types of dosages invariably lower TSH below the bottom of the TSH reference range, i.e. TSH is supressed. T3-Only also suppresses FT4 below the bottom of its range. Whereas, FT3 is often at the top of its reference range, or well above it, when symptom relief is achieved. This latter point really causes alarm for a lot of doctors! Current medical practice would suggest that these patients were hyperthyroid, or even thyrotoxic. They are thought to be vulnerable to heart attacks or bone loss. However, patients with lab results like these do not have the slightest indication of any over-dosing of T3.

Current FT3 reference ranges are developed from analysing a wide range of mostly T4-treated, in-range-TSH thyroid patients. These **FT3 population ranges** are definitely not representative of those on T3-Only, and are therefore of little use when managing a T3-Only dosage. See Chapter 14, for a powerful argument that shows why **the current FT3 reference range is not applicable to those on T3-Only**.

The other reason for **not** being constricted by lab test results is that a T3 dosage change can alter symptoms and signs rapidly. If symptoms and signs change a lot with a T3 dosage change, sometimes you need to be able to quickly adjust your T3 dosage. There is rarely enough time to get more lab tests done, even if they provided any insight (which they usually do not on T3-Only). Lab test results are also highly dependent on when the blood was drawn relative to the time of the last T3 dose. Labs are of no value in providing insight about 1 dose, which is a part of a 3-4 per day multi-dose regime. Labs are just not sensitive enough measures to allow anyone to carefully craft a safe T3 dosage that relieves symptoms.

So, what can be used to assess dosing in this case? The proven answer is symptoms and signs. These can be used in a very effective and systematic way to tailor each divided dose in terms of its size and timing. The result is an individually tailored T3 dosage that resolves symptoms and never causes over-stimulation. This individualised T3 dosage is likely to have 3 or 4 doses. Each of these could be of different sizes. The timings between them could also vary.

The *Recovering with T3* book explains the process to titrate the T3 dosage in detail.

## OTHER IMPORTANT BACKGROUND INFORMATION

The half-life of T3 is an interesting one to discuss. It is thought to be around 24 hours. When a T3 dose is taken, it is absorbed quite quickly, and then gets to work on raising metabolism very quickly after that.

Most thyroid patients on T3-Only find that the effects of a T3 dose can be felt rapidly. This can be within 30 minutes to 1 hour. I would certainly expect the effects to be felt within 2 hours. I do not know if the fast acting effects are non-genomic, or genomic, or a mixture. I just know that they are very real. It could be largely the effect on the mitochondria that can be experienced so quickly (non-genomic). More research is required.

Peak effects are often in the 2-4 hour period after the dose. The T3 dose typically begins to wear off somewhere in the 4-8 hour region. These effects vary somewhat by person. Consequently, as a practical guide to using T3, the half-life of T3 in the bloodstream is of no use in dosing decisions. I also suspect that only some of the T3 makes it into the cells and becomes active there.

T3 does not need to be taken on an empty stomach. I recommend simply chewing up the T3 dose and swallowing it.

3 T3 doses per day are the most common. It is common to take these doses: first thing in the morning, late morning/lunchtime, and finally, late afternoon. It is recommended that T3 is *not* used late in the evening, as often this can coincide with lower cortisol levels, and cause higher heart rate, anxiety and problems sleeping. For those with hypocortisolism, CT3M can be considered (see later in the chapter).

When T3 starts to be used, it will begin to lower your TSH. T3 medication lowers TSH far more than T4 medication. This, in turn, will lower native thyroid production and lower T4 to T3 conversion of your circulating T4. Because of this, T3 doses need to be raised slowly and carefully if the patient is to feel any real positive effect and remain safe. Changes need to be very small and un-dramatic. In some cases, increasing too quickly can, make the patient's existing T4 convert more effectively, and then they can feel extremely hyperthyroid. So, caution, caution, caution needs to be the mantra when managing T3-Only dosing.

In many cases, T3-Only relieves symptoms only at the point when the T3 dosage is close to suppressing the TSH, and FT4 and rT3 levels decline. Sometimes, there is a need for total

TSH suppression and near zero FT4 and rT3 before a significant therapeutic improvement occurs. This is my own situation, and I have seen the same thing with many other thyroid patients. It may be that you are one of those people too. Only when FT4 drops to near zero, and rT3 is virtually zero, do some people improve. Testing TSH can determine if you are on the way to this. However, having a low, or suppressed TSH does not mean that the T3 dosage is ideally adjusted to relieve all symptoms. More work on dosing may be needed.

Total daily TSH-suppressive doses of T3 vary by individual. They can be as low as 30 mcg per day but often are between 40 mcg and 50 mcg of T3. In a few people, it takes more T3 than this to fully suppress TSH.

As soon as T3-Only begins to be used, your own FT4 and rT3 ought to begin to reduce. However, for many T3-Only patients, they only get symptom relief when there is very low FT4 and rT3. This only begins to occur once the TSH-suppressive dosage has been reached. *Once the T3 dosage reaches that point, due to the T4 half-life, it can still take a further 8-12 weeks for FT4 and rT3 to reduce to a very low level. Patience is needed*.

A sound process for managing T3 doses, and being safe at all times, is essential - the *Recovering with T3* book provides this.

T3 medication must be taken at least an hour or more before any calcium or iron supplement. If any iron or calcium supplement is taken, leave at least 4 hours clear before taking the T3 medication.

Lots of small T3 doses tend not to be effective, e.g. taking 8 doses of 5 mcg of T3 is far less likely to raise metabolism compared to: a 15-mcg dose, and another 15-mcg dose followed by a 10-mcg dose. I am not entirely sure what the biochemistry of this is. In *Recovering with T3,* I explain that each T3 dose needs to be sufficient to get enough T3 into the cells and bind with the thyroid receptors in the cell nuclei and mitochondria. I suspect that only some of the T3 in a swallowed dose becomes effective within the cell nuclei and mitochondria. In any event, small doses do *not* tend to work well.

I will talk a little about dosing of T3 here. But the complete protocol may be found within *Recovering with T3.* There is a lot to know about T3 before using it. It requires diligence and a systematic approach, if you wish to find a well-tolerated, effective and safe dosage that never, at any time, causes over-stimulation. T3-Only is harder to use than the other therapies. But sometimes, it is the only one that will relieve symptoms, and then it can work wonders.

## STRATEGIES TO GET A TRIAL OF T3-ONLY

This can be difficult. It often relies upon finding a good and sympathetic doctor or endocrinologist. I do recommend that you reach out early to at least identify such a person and do not wait until you have discovered that the other treatments do not work. Join forums and talk to other patients. Quite often, other patients have recommendations of doctors or endocrinologists who are not stuck within the dogma that exists at present regarding T3-Only.

You could also consider getting the DIO2 gene tested. **Regenerus Labs** do provide the **DIO2** mutation test (which is the most important one of the two). Other companies may provide genetic testing, which will reveal both **D1 and D2 deiodinase gene defects**. However, you will need to check whether the company includes this information in its raw genome data - some do and some do not. If you can prove that you have a faulty gene that affects T4 to T3 conversion, this might help your case. Giving your doctor a copy of the Watts Study might be helpful.

If you have lost thyroid tissue through a thyroidectomy or through Hashimoto's thyroiditis, you will also have lost a substantial amount of T4 to T3 conversion. The thyroid gland converts more T4 than any other tissue. Making this point to your doctor may also help to persuade them to allow a trial of T3-Only.

Persistent hypocortisolism may also respond well to T3-Only therapy, as T3-Only stimulates the HP system far more than any other treatment.

Some thyroid patients who are tired of remaining ill and realise that a trial of T3-Only could provide a solution to their poor health, take matters more into their own hands, e.g. they begin to self-medicate with T3. I am not going to support or condone this. All I will say is that it is simply not good enough for so many doctors to condemn fellow human beings to permanent ill health, that could cost them their career and their family, through being too rigid in their thinking. The research is starting to become available to support a more flexible, caring and effective approach to treating all classes of hypothyroidism.

## START TRACKING SYMPTOMS AND SIGNS

I have already suggested that you begin to track symptoms and signs prior to taking any thyroid medication at all. This way, you will have a baseline, pre-treatment level. Comparisons can then be made to see how your treatment is progressing. I described how to do this in Chapter 13.

With T3-Only, it is best to do sets of readings when you wake, just before a daytime T3 dose and 2-3 hours after a T3 dose, plus one set in the evening. It can seem like a lot of work but it helps the process to go smoothly. From these sets of readings, you can see the effect of each daytime dose of T3. As the doses begin to be effective, changes in body temperature, heart rate, BP, and, importantly, symptoms can occur.

Take more readings if things begin to get confusing or worrying. Making careful notes and keeping them will be very useful indeed. You will be able to assess progress and watch out for problems. You will be able to summarise changes to your doctor and discuss the next steps.

## SWAPPING TO T3-ONLY

The process will be the same whatever thyroid medication you have been taking.

All T4-based medication is stopped. I prefer to leave one or more days without thyroid medication, and then allow some level of hypothyroid symptoms to develop before commencing T3-Only. This is because when T3 is given, it can sometimes cause an improvement in conversion that can make the patient hyperthyroid. Then the starting dosage is begun.

## STARTING DOSE OF T3-ONLY

Always start low on T3-Only. A low starting dosage of 2-3 doses of 5 mcg each is advisable. Your tolerance to the T3 can then be assessed. If you have not had cortisol tested, please consider starting even lower than this. Some people who are obviously hypothyroid can start a little higher, e.g. 3 doses of 10 mcg, 5 mcg, 5 mcg (as long as cortisol levels are fine). Clinical judgement needs to be used in deciding the starting dose, taking into account symptoms and signs, and the thyroid medication that you have been taking previously.

Starting low and raising the dosage slowly is the safest way of doing it. This is a long-distance race, not a sprint. Rushing will cause problems.

Try to keep exactly the same dose times each day, until you decide that you have to change them based on symptoms and signs.

## WHEN TO INCREASE/DECREASE, BY HOW MUCH AND TO WHICH DOSE?

Chapter 13 discusses all the most relevant information that can be used in driving decisions on when to make a T3-Only dosage change.

I recommend no change to the T3 dosage more often than every 4-5 days. Remember T3 is fast acting and does not take weeks to build up like T4-based meds.

Only ever change one dose, or the timing of one dose at a time.

Try to keep exactly the same dose times each day, until it is decided that a timing needs to change based on symptoms and signs.

Try not to add or remove more than a quarter of a T3 tablet (5 or 6.25 mcg) during any dosage change. Sometimes an even smaller change of 2.5 mcg might be desirable.

Assess the effect of the change compared to the symptoms/signs of the previous dosage.

Try to get to a point within 2-4 of weeks, where each dose is at least 10 mcg with perhaps the third dose being a little lower. These are unlikely to be therapeutic doses, but it does avoid small doses that do not usually work well.

Always be prepared to reverse the change if there is confusion.

Very often individual doses of between 10 and 25 mcg are found to be effective, with the largest ones usually occurring earlier in the day. T3 doses need to be built up slowly.

Changes to T3 dosing can sometimes be done every 4-5 days at the start when the dosage is very low. Later on, less frequent changes are more sensible.

I mentioned in Chapter 4, the genomic effects of T3 in the cell nuclei could take weeks or months to fully occur. This can be thought of as restructuring or reprogramming the genes. So, it sometimes takes patience in between increases, especially when the dosage is closer to a therapeutic level. The body needs the time to adjust.

***Please read the Recovering with T3 book for more details.*** Using T3-Only can be tricky. You need to be armed with as much information as possible to guide you and your doctor. It is unlikely that your doctor is going to be able to review your symptoms and signs and help you with every single dosing change. These changes need to be more frequent than T4-based medication. You will not be able to wait one month between changes in T3-dosage. Even two weeks would be pushing it. So, waiting for a doctor's appointment each time, is not going to be very effective, and will be likely to leave you feeling very hypothyroid.

Note - even if TSH is fully suppressed, there will be some remaining, basal level of thyroid gland secretion of thyroid hormones. However, the effect of thyroid medication is that gradually, over time, this basal secretion will reduce. So, the thyroid medication level may need to be increased slightly as time goes on.

## WHEN SHOULD A FULL THYROID PANEL BE REPEATED?

The answer to this is: **only when you have to**. It will not help you or your doctor with dosing decisions - as discussed above. However, checking very occasionally that FT3 is rising and FT4 & rT3 & TSH are all falling might confirm what you are seeing in symptoms and signs.

*If your doctor insists on thyroid blood tests, they must always be done first thing in the morning prior to the first dose of the day of thyroid medication. This includes any CT3M dose if you are using CT3M.*

## SYMPTOMS AND SIGNS WHEN T3-ONLY DOSAGE IS IDEAL

Please refer back to Chapter 13 & 14 for more details - these are just the main highlights that are likely to be present when your T3-Only dosage is optimal:

- You should feel well and have relief from all hypothyroid symptoms.
- Your body temperature should be normal for you  - see Chapter 13.
- Heart rate should be normal for you.
- Blood pressure should be normal for you.
- Note: the important thing is how the labs and symptoms adjust during treatment with respect to each other. Every individual is unique in terms of where their levels will sit when symptoms are relieved. See Chapter 14 for more details.
- TSH could be near the bottom of the range or suppressed below it (but remember this is not always the case for some people, and it is not a goal of the treatment). It takes time to slowly build up to a TSH suppressive dose of T3-Only.
- FT4 is very likely to be near the bottom of the reference range or totally suppressed near zero.
- FT3 is very likely to be at the top of the reference range, or well over the top of it. Remember the reference range for FT3 is the one used to manage patients on T4-Only therapy and should not be used to constrain T3 dosage for patients on T3-Only.
- RT3 will be zero or near zero or extremely low on T3-Only treatment. It takes time to build up to a TSH-suppressive dose of T3 (usually 40, or 50 mcg or more of T3).  At that point rT3 falls and will reduce to an extremely low level, over many weeks.

## BACKGROUND ON THE CIRCADIAN T3 METHOD (CT3M)

In Chapter 7, I described the 24-hour circadian relationship of cortisol to the thyroid hormones. If cortisol is mildly low, CT3M could be tried. In cases of severe hypocortisolism, you should be referred to an endocrinologist for further investigations.

In essence, CT3M begins by taking the first T3 dose of the day 1.5 hours before getting out of bed in the morning. This requires a bedside alarm to be set each night. The CT3M dose is taken and you go back to sleep. Ideally, all of this happens without turning on a light. Symptoms and signs are tracked over the coming days. If hypocortisolism is still suspected, the CT3M dose can either be moved 30 minutes earlier, or it can be increased by a small amount. The results are assessed and the last change can be reversed if it did not work. Symptoms and signs during the daytime provide the feedback. At some point, re-testing cortisol will be needed.

The CT3M dose can be moved as far back as 4 hours before the time that you get up in the morning, occasionally a little earlier than this. The CT3M dose sizes most commonly effective are between 15 and 25 mcgs. Although, as ever, a few people do better with less and a few need more.

CT3M does not work well for all people. However, it can work incredibly well for some. So, if cortisol is low, but not severely low, it is well worth trying prior to considering taking adrenal glandulars or HC.

***When CT3M works well, it will raise cortisol levels throughout the entire day.*** I have seen this many, many times over the past 10 years.

Raising cortisol levels in this way is extremely unlikely to produce hypercortisolism (too much cortisol or cortisol-effect). Higher T3 levels will balance the higher cortisol levels. It is always about the balance between the active thyroid hormone T3 and cortisol.

For information on CT3M please read ***Recovering with T3*** and ***The CT3M Handbook.***

## WHAT TO SUSPECT IF THERE ARE PROBLEMS?

It would be very unusual for no problems at all to appear during any thyroid hormone replacement. Some problems may not be thyroid hormone related. Symptoms and signs (Chapter 13) will often provide clues as to what the problem is.

Some of the basic things that can be wrong during treatment are:

- Not yet being on a high enough T3 dosage - being overly slow at increasing it, or perhaps being restricted by your doctor if he adheres to TSH or FT3 limits.
- Not absorbing the T3 properly, or not absorbing enough of it. Begin to suspect this if there is no symptomatic response during the day after the increased T3 doses. Lab testing may also help to confirm this is happening. Low stomach acid or gut issues could have a bearing in this case, as can taking the thyroid hormone too close to calcium or iron.
- Too much T3 thyroid hormone. Usually caused by trying to get to a therapeutic dosage too quickly. One would think that this would be easy to identify but sometimes, other issues

cause the same symptoms. However, a combination of both symptoms and signs ought to be able to identify excess T3. Sometimes other issues such as hypocortisolism or low iron can masquerade as too much T3. Stepping back down in dosage for a while is always a possibility.

- Trying to use only one dose per day of T3 rather than divided doses can also cause big issues. This is not a physiological replacement method.
- Not tracking symptoms and signs can mean you are missing some fluctuations that could tell you much about your dose sizes and their timings. It is essential on T3-Only to put the effort in to track symptoms and signs and be very systematic. It will not work without this.
- Hypocortisolism, low iron, low B12, low folate, low vitamin D, or issues with some other nutrient or condition may interfere with treatment and cause symptoms similar to the effects of either low or high thyroid hormone. Consequently, some or all of the pre-treatment tests could be run again.
- Chapters 20, 21 and 22 provide further ideas, if all other issues have been totally ruled out.
- Sometimes, with all the will in the world, T3-Only may not be right for an individual.

Your doctor and you will have to work out which is the most likely and test that hypothesis. Further lab tests might have to be run, e.g. a cortisol saliva test for hypocortisolism. If cortisol is low, investigations might need to be done to find out why and correct it.

### WHAT TO DO WHEN YOU FEEL WELL

When you have full symptom relief, your task is not yet done. You need to make a very clear record of:
- All symptom improvements in as much detail as you can, so that you can compare if things change.
- All signs that you can measure now in good health - body temperature, heart rate, blood pressure.
- All signs related to test results now - vitamins, minerals, etc.
- Thyroid lab results now - TSH, FT4, FT3, and rT3.
- In particular, please pay close attention to how the relationships of the thyroid labs have changed from when you felt ill, to now when you feel well. If you can see these from the results, you will recognise what works for you as an individual. If things drift out of balance in the future, you will be able to recognise this far more easily.

On T3-Only your thyroid lab results will be very unlike the lab results on any of the other treatments. They are unlikely to useful in making dosage decisions. However, this chapter gives you some idea of what to expect when a thyroid panel is run.

### T3-ONLY AND THE HEART, BONES, PREGNANCY, BRAIN AND NEED FOR T4

There is much misinformation, fear and rumour mongering about the effect of T3-Only. Some doctors get concerned over high FT3 levels, or no FT4 and suppressed TSH. Some patients remain in permanent ill-health because they are not allowed any further increases in T3. In the worst cases, I have heard of patients' T3 prescriptions being stopped altogether!

The evidence for any long-term **heart** problems or **bone** loss issues was dismissed by a 20-year observational study of patients using T3 - see **reference 3** in Resources. Anecdotally, I have witnessed evidence that supports improved bone density and better cardiovascular health with T3-Only. Any thyroid hormone therapy when badly dosed (low or high) can cause problems. T3-Only is no exception and should not get singled out.

As for the view that T3-Only is unsafe during **pregnancy**, I personally do not believe this. No research has actually occurred for women going through pregnancy on T3-Only. Moreover, I know of many women on T3-Only who have given birth to healthy babies, that have developed into healthy, happy and bright young children. A doctor might insist that a pregnant woman switch to a T4-based medication, but this may well make her very ill, which can be harmful to the foetus. A foetus begins to make its own thyroid hormone at 12 weeks and is self-sufficient at around 18-20 weeks. So a pragmatic compromise could be to take some T4-based medication, alongside the existing T3 medication, during the first 20 weeks of pregnancy. The T4 medication could then be withdrawn, if the mother is not feeling well on it. Please do your own research on this though. The above are merely my own views.

There has also been a lot of misinformation on the Internet and in other books that state that the **brain** cannot use T3-Only. All I will say on that is that thyroid patients using T3-Only are healthy, fit and happy and new research squashes that argument - **see reference 4**.

Doctors and some thyroid patients sometimes state that T4 has unique effects and it must also be taken. T4 does bind to receptors at the cell membrane. However, when T3-Only is used, the higher concentration of T3 also allows it to bind there; thus T3 fulfils the functions of both T4 and T3. There is no loss of any capability, which is why so many on T3-Only feel well. See my blog post in **reference 5** in Resources for more details.

With proper research, much of the misinformation and misplaced fear would vanish.

## HOW DO YOU SWITCH BRAND OF` T3 MEDICATION

You may occasionally be forced to deal with a new supplier of your medication. I recommend that at first, you only switch your last dose of the day to the new brand. This will allow you to assess its effect. Switching all doses in one-go would be foolhardy.

It is also important to be aware that not all preparations of the same medications are equal. Some are stronger or weaker than others. Some have different fillers and binders. I am not going to go into detail about this here, but changing from a medication that works well, to a new one, needs to be handled carefully. Assessing the difference by only changing one dose allows you to do a proper comparison. You may have to adjust the dose size of the new medication to something slightly different to your previous medication.

I have not put this section in the other treatment chapters because it applies to the other medications to a lesser extent.

## TRY TO AVOID PITFALLS & ROADBLOCKS

There are more pitfalls & roadblocks possible within treatment itself than in any other aspect of recovering from hypothyroidism. They are too numerous to list.

If you have a supportive doctor and can work in partnership with them, you will be subject to far fewer pitfalls & roadblocks.

Tracking symptoms and signs at home will provide you with the data that will show whether progress is being made or not. It will guide you into making dose size and timing adjustments that will lead to an effective and safe T3 dosage that is unique to you and your needs. This information will also give your doctor some confidence that you are assessing yourself, and they should be reassured over the safety of the treatment.

Be prepared when you see your doctor at each appointment. This will help enormously.

Please do not let your doctor drive your treatment using TSH alone, or even FT3. Lab test-centric dosage management will not work for T3-Only.

If you need a friend or relative to help you negotiate with your doctor, then teach them about hypothyroidism, loan them this book, and have them see your doctor with you at each appointment. Consider writing a simple letter prior to each appointment so that you do not get stressed during the appointment and forget something important. Negotiate for what you need, and why you need it, within the letter.

Read the *Recovering with T3* book - the information in this chapter is only a fraction of what the book contains.

If you have hypocortisolism and want to use CT3M, read *The CT3M Handbook* too.

Get as armed with as much information as possible, waste no time with bad choices.

Worst case, if your doctor is dogmatic, does not take your needs on board, or is using thyroid labs only to attempt to manage your treatment, work hard to find a better one.

If you want to get well as quickly as possible, you will need to get involved and gain some control of your health.

## RESOURCES

Here is a list of essential reading for those considering T3-Only use:

1. *Recovering with T3* - Paul Robinson (The complete T3-Only treatment protocol for the safe and effective use of T3. It also introduces the Circadian T3 Method (CT3M) ).

2. *The CT3M Handbook* - Paul Robinson (Contains more information on correcting hypocortisolism using T3 medication).

3. *Safety review of liothyronine use: a 20 year observational follow up study* - E. Soto-Pedre, G. Leese -http://www.endocrine-abstracts.org/ea/0038/ea0038OC5.6.htm

4. *T4 is NOT Needed in the Brain in Adults* - http://recoveringwitht3.com/blog/t4-not-needed-brain-adults-new-research-backs-t3-users-experience

5. *T3 is the main active thyroid hormone* - http://recoveringwitht3.com/blog/t3-main-active-thryoid-hormone

# Chapter 19

## T4/T3 Treatment

I have already discussed T4-Only treatment and T3-Only treatment. This chapter is about using a combination of T4 and T3. I am going to call this T4/T3 treatment.

### WHY CHOOSE THIS TREATMENT?

I think that the most obvious reason is that T4/T3 might be more palatable to a doctor, than offering NDT or T3-Only treatments. For some patients, it might also be possible to get symptom relief with only a little T3 added to the T4 medication.

T4/T3 also offers the opportunity to control the ratio of T4:T3, whereas with NDT the ratio of T4:T3 is fixed.

In the NDT treatment chapter, I stated that having some T3 in the mix provides more stability in the TSH and thyroid hormone system. The addition of T3 brings a much-needed stability to the entire system - this is a big advantage of T4/T3 treatment over T4-Only. See *reference 5* in Resources at the end of the chapter (only the abstract is available as I write this).

The final reason for someone ending up on T4/T3 is that some doctors are uncomfortable with their patients being on T3-Only and having no T4 in their bodies. I think this is a misplaced concern, but some patients do end up on a therapeutic dosage of T3, with a little T4 added. If your doctor is nervous about the T4/T3, take a copy of *reference 6* to them.

### HOW I WILL HANDLE THIS CHAPTER

I have already discussed T4-Only, NDT and T3-Only therapy. There is a great deal of information in those chapters that can be applied to T4/T3 treatment. I do not intend to repeat all of that. I will just outline the main options for T4/T3 use.

I am going to propose two approaches for using T4/T3, and only go into detail with one of them. To attempt to cover more than one approach would make this chapter too complicated to read.

### TWO APPROACHES FOR T4/T3 TREATMENT

I will assume that the starting point to using T4/T3 treatment is the same for both approaches. I will assume that you are already on a T4-Only dosage, but have not achieved full relief of symptoms, and this T4-Only dosage has been optimised as much as possible.

- *Approach 1* - keep on the same T4-Only dosage as at present until symptoms and signs show that it needs to be lowered or increased. Add 2.5-5 mcg of T3 at a time, splitting it into 2 or 3 divided doses of T3, with a weighting usually towards the morning. This is the approach I will discuss in more detail in the rest of the chapter. I think it is the simplest one for T4/T3 treatment.

- *Approach 2* - switch from T4-only to a 4:1 ratio of T4:T3, and use 2 or 3 divided doses, and small increments - very similar to NDT Treatment. This would mean the smallest unit of T4/T3 would be 20 mcg of T4 with 5 mcg of T3. This would be equivalent to the 1/2-grain units of NDT described in Chapter 17. The process of swapping over and raising doses would be exactly the same as for NDT. I will not explore this approach, as the 4:1 ratio is somewhat arbitrary and is unlikely to represent the actual human thyroid gland production ratio of T4:T3 - see Chapter 4 for more information on this.

**The rest of the chapter ONLY discusses Approach 1.**

### TYPICAL FINAL DAILY DOSAGE OF T4/T3

A typical final replacement dose of T4 and T3 could be highly variable. It depends on how much T3 was required and whether the T4 had to be lowered. It is impossible to say. NDT medication for adults is frequently between 2 and 5 grains. In T4/T3 terms this would be equivalent to 80 mcg of T4 with around 20 mcg of T3, up to 200 mcg of T4 with 50 mcg of T3 (at the extreme end). I expect a dosage somewhere in the middle is more likely - 140 mcg of T4 with up to 35 mcg of T3. However, some people might find they can do very well with a much smaller dose of T3, e.g. perhaps as little as only adding 5 or 10 mcg of T3. Others may have to reduce T4 significantly. Consequently, it is hard to suggest a final dosage expectation.

### OTHER IMPORTANT BACKGROUND INFORMATION

The T4 content of the T4/T3 has a half-life. This is the time it takes for half of the amount of the T4 in the blood to be eliminated. The half-life of T4 is 6-7 days for a healthy person, and 9-10 days for someone with hypothyroidism, whose metabolism is slower than a healthy person. The bottom line is that it takes 8-12 weeks for total stability of the FT4 level in the bloodstream. However, after 4-6 weeks much of this stabilising has already occurred.

T4/T3 can be taken on an empty stomach or not. However, if you have any concerns about absorption, taking it on an empty stomach 30-60 minutes before food would be safer.

When T3 is added, TSH will fall. This will potentially cause the same pattern as for the other T4 based therapies. You may feel better after an increase in T3, only to find that some days later you feel just the same as you did before the raise. The effect of TSH on conversion has already been explained. Patience may be needed as the doses of T3 and T4 are adjusted, TSH is lowered, and this mechanism ceases to be a problem.

Both T4 and T3 medication must be taken at least an hour or more before any calcium or iron supplement. If any iron or calcium supplement is taken, leave at least 4 hours clear before taking the thyroid medication.

See the other two T4-based therapies for more information (Chapters 15 & 16).

## START TRACKING SYMPTOMS AND SIGNS

I am suggesting that you begin to track symptoms and signs prior to starting to add any T3 medication at all. This way, you will have a baseline, pre-treatment level. Comparisons can then be made to see how your treatment is progressing. I described how to do this in Chapter 13. You will be able to summarise changes to your doctor and discuss the next steps.

## STARTING T3 DOSE TO BE ADDED TO EXISTING T4 MEDICATION

A reasonable start would be to add 5 mcg of T3, and to take it with the morning dose of T4, although 10 mcg might be tolerated (in which case splitting that into two divided doses - morning and mid-afternoon would be sensible). Much would depend on symptoms and signs and how much of a boost you require. If your symptoms were minor, you may get away with only 2.5 mcg morning and afternoon.

## WHEN TO INCREASE/DECREASE, BY HOW MUCH AND TO WHICH DOSE?

Chapter 13 discusses all the most relevant information that can be used when assessing a dosage change and how much of a change to make.

The recommendation is to use 5-mcg increments of T3. With T3, changes can usually be made once a week quite safely, if the increases are only 5 mcg at a time.

Symptoms and signs can be used to determine when to take the T3. Timing of T3 doses can be crucial. Once someone is at, or over, 10 mcg of T3 total for the day, I would definitely suggest using 2 divided doses, i.e. 5 mcg + 5 mcg. One of these should be taken in the morning with the T4 medication and one in the mid to late afternoon.

A balance of T3 more heavily weighted towards the morning would be better. Consequently, if you were already on a 5-mcg morning T3 dose and a 5-mcg afternoon T3 dose, the next 5-mcg increment ought to be added to the morning dose.

Symptoms and signs can guide the size of doses, their timings, and whether 3 divided doses would be better than 2.

It is possible that, due to the results of a thyroid panel, or symptoms and signs, the T4 portion of the T4/T3 dosage needs to be adjusted. It would depend on how well the T4 was converting. If it is not converting well, lowering the T4 dosage might be advisable.

When a final dose that relieves symptoms appears to be in sight, waiting longer between dosage changes is sensible - perhaps 8-12 weeks, if the T4 level has been adjusted, or 2 weeks if a T3 dose has been adjusted.

I mentioned in Chapter 4, the genomic effects of T3 in the cell nuclei could take weeks or months to fully occur. This can be thought of as restructuring or reprogramming the genes. So, it sometimes takes patience in between increases, especially when the dosage is closer to a therapeutic level. The body needs the time to adjust.

The effect of taking thyroid medication is that gradually any basal thyroid secretion will reduce. So, the thyroid medication may need to be increased slightly as time goes on.

## WHEN SHOULD A FULL THYROID PANEL BE REPEATED?

Typically, these are repeated when there is a need to understand what might be happening. It might be every 8-12 weeks. Note: when T3 is added to T4, this can lower conversion and decrease some FT3 and increase rT3.

A full thyroid panel including TSH, FT4, FT3 and rT3 would be best. *A minimal set of TSH, FT4 and FT3 ought to be run though.* If things are not progressing well you may begin to suspect conversion issues. In this case, getting FT3 and rT3 tested would be very helpful, even if you need to do this privately.

However, many doctors only repeat TSH. This is a huge issue. Ideally, a full thyroid panel, *combined with symptoms*, should be used to assess dosage changes. Please ensure FT3 is tested as part of the thyroid panel. See Chapter 14 for interpretation of a full thyroid panel when under treatment.

*Any thyroid blood test must always be done first thing in the morning, prior to the first dose of the day of thyroid medication. This includes any CT3M dose if you are using CT3M.*

## SYMPTOMS AND SIGNS WHEN T4/T3 DOSAGE IS IDEAL

Please refer back to Chapter 13 & 14 for more details - these are just the main highlights that are likely to be present when the T4/T3 dosage is optimal:

- You should feel well and have relief from all hypothyroid symptoms.
- Your body temperature should be normal for you - see Chapter 13.
- Your heart rate should be normal for you.
- Blood pressure should be normal for you.
- Note: the important thing is how the labs and symptoms adjust during treatment with respect to each other. Every individual is unique in terms of where their levels will sit when symptoms are relieved. See Chapter 14 for more details.
- TSH could be near the bottom of the range or suppressed below it (but remember this is not always the case for some people, and it is not a goal of the treatment).
- FT4 could be mid-range or above (this is not as important as FT3). In some cases, good T4 to T3 conversion may mean FT4 is below mid-range. There is no need to try to get FT4 high in the range (where it is more likely to create too much rT3).
- FT3 is very likely to be elevated into the top half of the range or near the very top.
- RT3 should be very low to mid-range at the most. RT3 may be extremely low if the T3 to T4 ratio is high in favour of T3.

## THE CIRCADIAN T3 METHOD (CT3M)

In the case where there is hypocortisolism, some of the T3 content could be used to implement the CT3M protocol. This sometimes works, even with T4/T3 medication. It might be that a good proportion of the T3 content needs to be used for CT3M, but the effect of more cortisol could make the daytime thyroid hormones work far better. Find out a little more about CT3M in Chapter 18 (T3 Treatment), and in the ***Recovering with T3*** and ***The CT3M Handbook.***

## WHAT TO SUSPECT IF THERE ARE PROBLEMS?

It would be very unusual for no problems at all to appear during any thyroid hormone replacement. Some problems may not be thyroid hormone related. Symptoms and signs (Chapter 13) will often provide clues as to what the problem is.

Some of the basic things that can be wrong during treatment are:

- Not being on a high enough T3 (or possibly T4) dose yet - being overly slow at increasing it. Due to the effect of lowering TSH affecting conversion, this can cause you to stay hypothyroid for a while, or even get more so. Tracking symptoms and signs will help to avoid this.
- Not absorbing the T4/T3 properly, or not absorbing enough of it. Lab testing may also help to confirm this is happening. Low stomach acid or gut issues could have a bearing in this case, as can taking the thyroid hormone too close to calcium or iron.
- Not converting enough T4 to T3 (testing FT3 will show this, and testing FT3 and rT3 will show it further). If the cause of the poor conversion cannot be found and corrected, switching to T3-Only may be necessary.
- The T4 content might need to be reduced significantly in favour of more T3 content.
- Too much thyroid hormone. Usually caused by trying to get to a therapeutic dosage too quickly. One would think that this would be easy to identify but sometimes, other issues cause the same symptoms. However, a combination of both symptoms and signs, including full thyroid labs, ought to be able to identify excess thyroid hormone. Stepping back down in dosage for a while is always a possibility.
- Trying to use only one dose per day of T3 can also cause big issues. That dose can have far too much T3 content.
- Not tracking symptoms and signs, and only going on thyroid labs to guide dosage changes.
- Hypocortisolism, a low vitamin or mineral or some other issue that is interfering with treatment, and causing symptoms similar to the effects of either low or high thyroid hormone. Consequently, some or all of the pre-treatment tests could be run again.
- Chapters 20, 21 and 22 provide further ideas, if all other issues have been totally ruled out.
- Sometimes, with all the will in the world, T4/T3 may not be right for an individual.

Your doctor and you will have to work out which is the most likely and test that hypothesis. Further lab tests might have to be run, e.g. a cortisol saliva test for hypocortisolism. If cortisol is low, investigations might need to be done to find out why and correct it.

If the T4/T3 treatment cannot be made to fully resolve symptoms, swapping to another thyroid treatment ought to be considered.

## WHAT TO DO WHEN YOU FEEL WELL

When you have full symptom relief, your task is not yet done. You need to make a very clear record of:

- All symptom improvements in as much detail as you can, so that you can compare if things change.
- All signs that you can measure now in good health - body temperature, heart rate, blood pressure.
- All signs related to test results now - vitamins, minerals, etc.
- Note: the important thing is how the labs and symptoms adjust during treatment with respect to each other. Every individual is unique in terms of where their levels will sit when symptoms are relieved. See Chapter 14 for more details.
- Thyroid lab results now - TSH, FT4, FT3, and rT3.
- In particular, please pay close attention to how the relationships of the thyroid labs have changed from when you felt ill, to now when you feel well. If you can see these from the results, you will recognise what works for you as an individual. If things drift out of balance in the future, you will be able to recognise this far more easily.
- The FT3 to FT4 ratio.

The balance of your thyroid lab results is going to be unique to you, and they may vary over time. This is what I talked about earlier in the book, when I explained that your own personal thyroid levels for good health are unique to you, and that they may have altered from when you had no thyroid issues. See *references 3 and 4* in Resources.

## TRY TO AVOID PITFALLS & ROADBLOCKS

There are more pitfalls & roadblocks possible within treatment itself than in any other aspect of recovering from hypothyroidism. They are too numerous to list.

If you have a supportive doctor and can work in partnership with them, you will be subject to far fewer pitfalls & roadblocks.

Tracking symptoms and signs at home will provide you with a lot of data that will show whether progress is being made or not. This will also reveal problems far sooner, and often more accurately, than a thyroid blood test panel.

Be prepared when you see your doctor at each appointment. This will also help.

Push to get a full thyroid panel when your blood tests are due to occur. Get copies of the results and record which lab did them. If you cannot get an rT3 test then look into doing FT3 and rT3 privately.

Please do not let your doctor drive your treatment using TSH alone, or even thyroid labs alone. Your symptoms and other signs are crucial in good clinical decision-making.

If you need a friend or relative to help you negotiate with your doctor, then teach them about hypothyroidism, loan them this book, and have them see your doctor with you at each appointment. Consider writing a simple letter prior to each appointment so that you do not get stressed during the appointment and forget something important. Negotiate for what you need, and why you need it, within the letter.

If you have tried T4/T3 and it does not work well, and no other issue can be found, a trial of T3-Only would be sensible. Consider, using the information in the T3-Only chapter to attempt to persuade your doctor. It may work.

Worst case, if your doctor is dogmatic, does not take your needs on board, or is using thyroid labs only to manage your treatment, work hard to find a better one.

If you want to get well as quickly as possible, you will need get involved and gain some control of your health.

If it does not look like even T4/T3 is going to work, do try to get a trial of T3-Only.

## RESOURCES

Here is a list of further reading for those who wish to find out more:

1. *Recovering with T3* - Paul Robinson. (See information on CT3M).
2. *The CT3M Handbook* - Paul Robinson. (More information on CT3M).
3. *Recent Advances in Thyroid Hormone Regulation: Toward a New Paradigm for Optimal Diagnosis and Treatment* - Hoermann, Midgley, Larisch, Dietrich. See: https://www.frontiersin.org/articles/10.3389/fendo.2017.00364/full
   (This paper talks about the need for a new paradigm of thyroid treatment that accepts that the relationship between TSH and thyroid hormones are individual, dynamic and can adapt, i.e. the current practice of simply looking at numbers that do, or do not, fit in the population ranges, is resulting in poor patient care).
4. *Narrow individual variations in serum T(4) and T(3) in normal subjects a clue to the understanding of subclinical thyroid disease* - Stig Anderson. See: https://academic.oup.com/jcem/article/87/3/1068/2846746
5. *Mathematical modeling of the pituitary-thyroid feedback loop: role of a TSH-T3-shunt and sensitivity analysis* - Berberich, Dietrich, Hoermann and Muller. See: https://www.frontiersin.org/articles/10.3389/fendo.2018.00091/abstract
   (The full article is not available yet, but this paper shows how T3 helps to stabilise the TSH-thyroid hormone system).
6. *Effects of Long-Term Combination LT4 and LT3 Therapy for Improving Hypothyroidism and Overall Quality of Life* - Tariq et al. See: https://www.ncbi.nlm.nih.gov/pmc/articles/PMC5965938/

# Chapter 20

## Dietary Considerations

I have been very lucky with respect to my response to food types. I eat quite simply, but I have never found the need to use a rigorous regime in order to feel well. When I have attempted a special type of diet, there has been no discernable benefit.

I eat 2 simple meals a day. I love vegetables and eat a balanced diet. I am 6 foot 1 inch (1.85 metres) tall, and my body mass index (BMI) is in the healthy range. I exercise virtually every single day (sit ups, weights, exercise bike). I play golf (badly) and very occasionally tennis (also badly these days). A lack of a particular diet is not hurting my ability to feel well, have good energy and enjoy my life.

However, I know that for some people, the foods that they eat, and the way in which these affect their systems is very important.

I remember many years ago, when I was first trying to learn about the causes of Hashimoto's thyroiditis, the phrase at the time was 'gluten-free'! Well, 'grain-free', and 'anti-candida' superseded this, then it was 'leaky-gut repair', and then 'Paleo' etc.

I do not believe there is a 'one size fits all' diet. I also know, for a fact, that I am absolutely no expert in this area - that much should be obvious by now! Yet, there still needs to be a small chapter in this book, which recognises that gut health, and the foods that some of us eat, will be important in our recovery. This will not apply to everyone, and it will not be the same solution for all.

These days, many people have a great deal of success with a dietary intake based on our stone-age ancestors. Paleo, Paleo-ketogenic and Stone-age diets are often discussed. I know some people who do feel significantly healthier on them. They have more energy, fewer health issues and, in some cases, have been able to reduce their thyroid hormone dosage.

### A note about eating disorders

There is a significant connection between eating disorders and hypothyroidism.

Unfortunately, untreated or incorrectly treated hypothyroidism can actually precipitate an eating disorder. This is because hypothyroidism commonly causes weight gain, which in some cases can be extreme or lifelong. This weight gain will not correlate with calories or the quality of the diet. In response to this, many start to restrict their diet. However, this restriction does not work very well and usually requires that the diet get stricter and stricter over time. Ultimately, the situation can spiral and an eating disorder may develop.

It is vital to understand that you do not have to be underweight to have an active eating disorder. Losing weight or even maintaining weight is often hard to do if you are not correctly treated for hypothyroidism. This latter point includes being on the right thyroid medication for you and on the right dosage. Other factors enabling the thyroid treatment to work would also need to have been addressed.

## Finally

I am not an expert in the area of diet myself. So, I am just going to leave a few references here as a starting point. You will need to make your own journey to discover if dietary considerations are going to be important to you or not:

## RESOURCES

Here is a list of some books on the subject of dietary considerations, gut health and why they might be important:

1. *The Paleo Thyroid Solution* - Elle Russe, with in-depth commentary from integrative physician Gary E. Foreman M.D.
2. *Practical Paleo* - Diane Sanfilippo, Bs, NC.
3. *The PK Cookbook* - Dr Sarah Myhill and Craig Robinson.
4. *Prevent and Cure Diabetes (Delicious diets not dangerous drugs)* - Dr Sarah Myhill and Craig Robinson.
5. *Sustainable Medicine* - Dr. Sarah Myhill (Chapter 3 in her book - The tools of the trade to correct and treat mechanisms of disease).
6. *Hashimoto's Thyroiditis* - Izabella Wentz, PharmD, FASCP. (Chapter 18 in her book - Diet for Hashimoto's).
7. *Wheat Belly* - William Davis, MD.
8. *Signs of an eating disorder* - https://www.nationaleatingdisorders.org/warning-signs-and-symptoms
9. *Health at Every Size* – Linda Bacon
10. *The Fat Nutritionist* - Michelle is a qualified dietician who specialises in eating disorder recovery - http://www.fatnutritionist.com

# Chapter 21

## Could Sex Hormones be a Problem?

There are very important connections between sex hormones, cortisol levels and the effectiveness of thyroid treatment. Hence, sex hormones deserve a chapter of their own.

The adrenal glands only produce a very small fraction of our sex hormones.

For men, this adrenal production of testosterone is so small compared to that produced by the testes that it is irrelevant. I have a section towards the end of the chapter entitled Men and Testosterone. Male patients could choose to skip straight to that section. Having said that, there is still useful information in the early parts of this chapter for a male patient.

For women, the situation can be very complex. Hence, this chapter focuses mostly on women, and in particular, on post-menopausal women, as the assessment and treatment of their sex hormones is far more straightforward.

For women who are still cycling, trying to fine-tune sex hormones can be highly problematic. Some cycling women do benefit from progesterone supplementation in the second half of their cycle to resolve symptoms like breast tenderness, heavy bleeding etc. However, my advice is to seek out the help of a specialist, if you are cycling and are having sex hormone issues.

### THE ADRENAL GLANDS & CORTISOL & SEX HORMONE PRODUCTION

There are complex interactions among all the hormones both within tissues and in the hypothalamic-pituitary system. This book does not have the scope to go into this very much.

Please refer back to Chapter 5 for a discussion of how the adrenal glands make their hormones. In this chapter, I will only be discussing sex hormones and the other adrenal hormones that have important relationships with them.

The adrenal cortex of each adrenal gland makes all of its hormones from cholesterol. Cholesterol is converted into pregnenolone, then into all other hormones including progesterone and 11-alpha hydroxy progesterone from which all the other adrenal steroids are made. See *reference 1* for a clear and comprehensive diagram that shows the hormone creation pathways. In addition to cortisol and aldosterone, the adrenal glands secrete some progesterone and androstenedione. Androstenedione can be converted in the peripheral tissues into estrone and from this into oestradiol (US spelling is estradiol). The adrenal glands secrete large amounts of DHEA and DHEAS. DHEA can be converted into both androgens and oestrogens within tissues throughout the body.

The adrenal production of progesterone in both men and women is only a tiny amount compared to that produced by the ovaries in a woman who is still cycling, during her luteal phase. Adrenal progesterone production is not controlled by the pituitary gland - it just occurs at very low constant level in both sexes. The progesterone production by the adrenals is of the same level in both women and men. After menopause the ovaries no longer make oestradiol and progesterone. So, the progesterone levels fall to the same low level as in men. The adrenal glands have the same structure and function in both sexes. So, it follows that low progesterone levels should not directly impact cortisol production in men or women, unless there was some associated HP dysfunction.

As mentioned in Chapter 5, the **adrenal glands only need sufficient ACTH stimulation and enough cholesterol to produce cortisol**, as long as there is no Addison's disease. With sufficient ACTH, higher serum progesterone levels should not be able to increase adrenal cortisol production. The addition of progesterone, or pregnenolone, is not able to directly increase cortisol production. Even in the presence of very low cholesterol levels, the adrenals continue to make sufficient cortisol and sex hormones - see **reference 5** in Resources.

Oestradiol is not secreted in significant amounts by the adrenal glands. It is made in the ovaries in cycling women and is produced within the peripheral tissues of both sexes from androstenedione, DHEA and testosterone.

Testosterone is made in the ovaries in cycling women and in the testes in men. A tiny amount of testosterone is secreted by the adrenal glands but it is small compared to the amount of testosterone made from androstenediol and DHEA in the peripheral tissues in both sexes.

ACTH production by the pituitary gland stimulates cortisol and DHEA production strongly.

When the ovaries fail to function in menopause, having run out of viable eggs, the pituitary secretes LH and FSH in very high amounts to try to stimulate ovarian function. LH and FSH remain at very high levels throughout menopause. In some women, the **loss of oestradiol, and the resultant very high LH and FSH levels may cause HP dysfunction**. This may affect ACTH production and cause a decrease in cortisol levels (or an increase in some cases). This is turn can affect thyroid hormone treatment, as already discussed many times. **In this one circumstance, supplementation with sex hormones may resolve any HP dysfunction, and help to restore healthy cortisol levels.**

## Sex hormones, cortisol and stress

Under stress, more ACTH is secreted by the pituitary gland. Therefore the adrenals make more cortisol, more DHEA and even aldosterone. The effect of continued stress can cause a change in the HP system - it becomes dysfunctional and stops making sufficient ACTH. Many studies show lower saliva cortisol levels in individuals with chronic stress, burn out and post-traumatic stress disorder. Perhaps the adrenal glands also become less sensitive to ACTH. The net result of continued stress is that less cortisol, DHEA and other hormones are produced within the adrenal glands. This is a pattern we see so many times in cortisol saliva test results. Initially, cortisol and DHEA can rise significantly, but eventually they fall. It has nothing to do with adrenal gland tiredness or fatigue - it is due to HP dysfunction after continued stress. Since it is possible for menopause to also cause HP dysfunction, through very high FSH and LH, post-menopausal women who are under stress, are in the worst position.

*Oestradiol, and to a lesser extent progesterone, can counteract cortisol-effect in the tissues.* The high oestradiol and progesterone levels in the luteal phase (second half of the menstrual cycle) can worsen an underlying hypocortisolism. This reduces cortisol-effect in the brain and other tissues and can cause the premenstrual syndrome and premenstrual dysphoric disorder. This is why, between ovulation and their menses, many women suffer from symptoms that are similar to hypocortisolism: fatigue, irritability, brain fog, poor sleep, etc. Since oestradiol counteracts cortisol strongly, many oestrogen dominance symptoms are actually due to hypocortisolism. Others are due to insufficient progesterone to balance the oestradiol, e.g. tender breasts, heavy bleeding, fluid retention. This interaction between oestradiol and cortisol explains why many women feel better in menopause - they no longer have so much oestradiol counteracting cortisol-effect.

## Menopause, sex hormones and cortisol

Menopause is the failure of major endocrine glands (the ovaries) and produces well-known symptoms and disorders. Insufficient oestradiol-effect in the tissues in menopause, causes hot flashes, vaginal dryness, insomnia, memory problems, osteoporosis, etc. The symptoms of menopause generally have little to do with cortisol, per se, except that hypocortisolism can cause hot flashes too. Women, who make more oestradiol after menopause, mostly from the conversion of DHEA and testosterone into oestradiol, have less severe oestradiol-deficiency symptoms. Obese women tend to have higher oestradiol levels, as fat contains aromatase, so they convert androgens (from the adrenals and remnant ovaries) into oestradiol more effectively. A few women do not require oestradiol replacement in menopause, but they almost all require progesterone to counteract/balance oestradiol's stimulatory effects in the uterus and breasts. Without sufficient progesterone levels, unopposed oestrogen-stimulation of the uterus and breasts causes cellular proliferation, which can promote the growth of any cancers that arise in these organs. Many women in menopause would also benefit from testosterone supplementation to restore youthful levels. Testosterone improves muscle strength and recovery time, reduces anxiety, and improves libido and sexual function.

Many women in menopause with hypocortisolism cannot tolerate oestradiol, as it counteracts cortisol, and worsens their hypocortisolism. Some women require cortisol supplementation in order to tolerate oestradiol supplementation. Progesterone's effects on cortisol are mixed and depend upon the woman. Progesterone is a partial agonist at the cortisol receptor. So, if cortisol is very low, progesterone can stimulate receptors and improve cortisol-effect. This explains why some women have better energy on progesterone supplementation. In other women who have higher but insufficient cortisol levels, progesterone can occupy cortisol receptors but not stimulate them sufficiently, resulting in an anti-cortisol-effect. It is also possible that with low oestradiol and low progesterone at menopause, some level of HP dysfunction can occur. Sex hormone supplementation restores a more youthful/healthy hormonal situation and in some women it can improve their hypocortisolism.

## Conclusions on sex hormones and the adrenals in post-menopausal women

The bottom line is that menopause is the failure of a major endocrine gland. It leaves women in a state of almost complete oestradiol deficiency - with much lower oestradiol levels than men! Menopause causes many problems for a woman's quality of life and long-term health. Stress can also be a huge factor, as it may lead to HP dysfunction and lower levels of cortisol, DHEA, oestradiol, progesterone and testosterone after menopause. Many post-menopausal women require supplementation of progesterone to maintain their well-being and their health. Some require progesterone, oestradiol, and testosterone supplementation to achieve this.

It may be near impossible for a post-menopausal woman to achieve her desired level of health and well-being, without addressing the low sex hormone issues.

## THERE ARE A FEW THINGS THAT CAN BE DONE

- Help to support the adrenals as much as possible.
- Find out if there is a sex hormone problem.
- Take steps if there is a sex hormone problem. At the very least, make a conscious decision over what you want to do, armed with proper data.

I will deal with each of the above in turn.

## SUPPORTING THE ADRENALS

There is no guarantee that this approach will help but it may be worth a try:

- Try to eat a cleaner diet to put less stress on the gut, e.g. less processed food, less sugar, trying a diet like Paleo etc.
- Supplements like B complex, magnesium and vitamin C can also help support the adrenals and immune system. I have already outlined a basic supplement regime in Chapter 12. There may be more specific nutritional supplements for the adrenals and sex hormones. You may have to do more of your own research into this.
- Try to limit both physical and mental stress, including strenuous exercise.
- Reduce or avoid alcohol and caffeine.
- Regular gentle exercise is a good idea.
- As mentioned earlier, the adrenal glands do not get fatigued or tired. In most cases, the adrenals work perfectly normally if there is sufficient cholesterol and ACTH

stimulation from the HP system, i.e. no HP-dysfunction. So, supplements etc. may not help a great deal.

## FINDING OUT IF THERE IS A SEX HORMONE PROBLEM POST-MENOPAUSE

Your symptoms will provide many clues about whether you have a sex hormone problem after you stop cycling or are post-menopausal.

*Low oestrogen* causes a range of problems: hot flashes, depression, fatigue, lower vaginal lubrication, mood swings, headaches, concentration problems, an increase in urinary tract infections due to thinning of the urethra. Low oestrogen will also tend to expose you to the risk of lower bone density.

*Low progesterone* causes headaches, mood changes, anxiety, depression, hot flashes, low sex drive. Progesterone is also needed to balance out oestrogen. If progesterone is too low in comparison to oestrogen; this is known as oestrogen dominance.

*Oestrogen dominance* causes breast tenderness, decreased sex drive, irritability, depression, bloating/water retention, fibrocystic breasts, weight/fat gain, hair loss, thyroid hormone dysfunction, brain fog, fatigue and insomnia.

Once your cycles have ceased, some of the symptoms alone could point to sex hormone problems. Verifying this through blood tests should be quite straightforward, as long as your doctor is willing to run the right tests.

If you have a competent doctor who fully understands sex hormones and sex hormone replacement, should it be required, interpreting the results of sex hormone blood tests should be straightforward. It does take some specialist knowledge. Simply looking at sex hormones and seeing if they fit within the lab ranges is not going to be sufficient. That should be of no surprise to you by now. Here are some background guidelines that may be helpful:

- Oestrogen is a collective term covering oestradiol, estrone and estriol. Usually, when a woman has oestrogen tested it is actually only oestradiol that is measured. However, some doctors recommend that after menopause, estrone also be tested, as it becomes more relevant than before menopause. Total oestrogen tests are not accurate enough.
- The following contains what are considered to be optimal levels. They will be different to the much wider reference ranges that will appear on lab test results.

### How to test sex hormones

The best way to do this is through *blood tests* for oestradiol, progesterone and testosterone. DHEAS and sex hormone binding globulin (SHBG) are also worth testing. Blood tests are usually more reliable.

If you are not supplementing hormones, saliva testing is also valid. *However, once supplementation of sex hormones has begun, only blood tests yield accurate information*.

*For non-cycling/post-menopausal women,* as long as you are *not* taking any form of hormone, the blood draw can happen at any time.

If you are on HRT or using some form of hormone replacement, leave *8-10 hours after your last dose/use of a sex hormone before the blood draw*.

## OPTIMAL SEX HORMONES - NON-CYCLING/POST-MENOPAUSAL WOMEN

These results are all based on *blood testing*. These are for guidance only, as if oestrogen or progesterone are low, the goals of any replacement is primarily symptom relief - not chasing numbers through blood testing. You should seek the help of a competent specialist, who may have different views on the optimal ranges and the treatment protocol.

### Optimal progesterone - non-cycling/post-menopausal women:

US units:             8-10 ng/mL

European units:       25-32 nmol/L

This is 35-45th percentile of the reference range for the Luteal phase in cycling woman.

Note: labs/doctors assume that the post-menopausal progesterone level will be significantly lower than this, e.g. < 0.6-3.0 nmol/L. However, the experience of patients, and doctors who specialise in bio-identical hormone replacement, is that women are often very symptomatic when their progesterone remains very low. Hence, the optimal level quoted above is a lot higher than what is shown on lab test results for a post-menopausal woman. The most important part of treating menopausal patients is the reduction and cessation of symptoms. As long as this is achieved, lower levels are acceptable, as long as they are in balance with oestrogen levels.

### Optimal Oestradiol (Estradiol) - non-cycling/post-menopausal women:

US units:             20-40 pg/mL

European units:       73-147 pmol/L

This is 36-73rd percentile of the reference range for post-menopausal oestradiol levels.

### Progesterone to Oestradiol Ratio - non-cycling/post-menopausal women:

Progesterone and oestradiol need to be balanced in an ideal ratio.

To calculate the progesterone to oestradiol ratio:

- Firstly, convert progesterone into the same units as oestradiol. You may have to Google a converter from one unit to the other to do this. This should make the progesterone number *a lot larger*.
- Secondly, once they are both in the same units, divide the progesterone number by the oestradiol number. This is the progesterone to oestradiol ratio.

The ideal ratio between progesterone and oestradiol should be *between 200:1 and 300:1*.

If the ratio is a lot less than this, the woman is still oestrogen dominant, regardless of whether or not oestrogen is low.

Here is a US units P/E ratio calculator: https://instacalc.com/779

Here is a European units P/E calculator: https://instacalc.com/36322

### SHBG (Sex Hormone Binding Globulin) - non-cycling/post-menopausal women

SHBG's job is to preferentially bind up Dihydrotestosterone (DHT), testosterone, androstenediol, oestradiol, and then estrone, in that order. DHEA, but not DHEAS, can bind weakly to SHBG. If SHBG is high, optimal levels of oestradiol may need to be higher for a patient to feel well and not experience low estrogen symptoms (hot flashes, incontinence, vaginal dryness, etc.).

Generally speaking, if SHBG is above optimal (100 nmol/L), the following levels of oestradiol may be acceptable, as a portion of the oestradiol is bound by SHBG:

- SHBG 100-130 nmol/L => oestradiol 110-125 pg/mL
- SHBG 130-160 nmol/L => oestradiol 125-140 pg/mL
- SHBG 160-190 nmol/L => oestradiol 140-155 pg/mL
- SHBG >190 nmol/L    => oestradiol 155-170 pg/mL

### Optimal total testosterone - non-cycling/post-menopausal women

US units:              28-38 ng/dL
European units:        1.0-1.32 nmol/L

Aiming to be mid-range or in the 3rd quartile would be ideal.

Free testosterone or free testosterone % are often referenced as a suitable measurement of testosterone levels in women. Typically, these serum levels should also be in the mid-range to 3rd quartile range or 2.10-3.20 pg/mL (US units) and 7-11 pmol/L (European). Healthy free testosterone % is 1.6-2.5% of total testosterone levels.

### DHEAS (DHEA-Sulfate)

DHEA is a master, or parent, hormone that the body changes into a hormone called androstenedione. Androstenedione is then converted into the major female and male hormones, testosterone and oestrogen. DHEAS contains a sulfate molecule, and more than 90% of the DHEA in your bloodstream exists in the form of DHEAS. The body produces DHEA primarily in the morning hours, and the kidneys secrete this DHEA very quickly. DHEAS, however, remains in your body much longer. For this reason, doctors use DHEAS levels to determine the blood level of the DHEA in your body. Low DHEAS can be a sign of adrenal dysfunction. High DHEAS may indicate the beginning stages of hypocortisolism.

*It is very important to be aware that DHEA is necessary to offset the catabolic effect of cortisol within the body. Healthy or high cortisol levels with low DHEA can be very damaging to the tissues.*

The reference range for DHEAS varies with age, e.g. in the US, an 18-year old has a range of 145-395 ug/dL, whereas for an over 40-year old it drops to 32-240 ug/dL.

The units also vary by country, e.g. in the UK, DHEAS is often measured in umol/L.

The following are still serum/blood measures (DHEAS can also be measured in saliva). *Please have the DHEAS test 12 hours following any daily dose of DHEA if it is being supplemented*.

### *Optimal DHEAS - non-cycling/post-menopausal women*

US units: 145-395 ug/dL
European units: 1.75-10.26 umol/L

DHEAS ought to be at mid-range to the higher end of the range to ensure good adrenal function on average over 24 hours, and to **offset the catabolic effects of cortisol on the body** (ageing, depressed immune system, inflammatory bowel issues, muscle loss etc.).

If someone has had low DHEAS for some time, re-introducing it can be tricky, because people become very sensitive to it. They have to reintroduce it very slowly, starting with just 2.5mg sublingually or vaginally. Eventually, after a month or two, it can be increased to 5mg daily. Swallowing DHEA produces more of the sulfate and may cause acne. Most women need only 2.5 to 12.5mg/day sublingually or vaginally.

## NEXT STEPS IF A NON-CYCLING/POST-MENOPAUSAL WOMAN HAS A SEX HORMONE PROBLEM

If there is an imbalance you will have choices to make. Not everyone chooses hormone replacement. Some people work on diet and lifestyle changes, hoping that these will correct the imbalances. For others, hormone replacement is an option, and can be very effective in resolving symptoms.

Please do seek out the help of a competent and experienced specialist.

### Goals of any sex hormone replacement after menopause

If you are a non-cycling/post-menopausal woman, and you are symptomatic, if one or more of the hormones is low compared to optimal post-menopausal levels, the goal would be to supplement to a point to resolve these issues.

Symptom relief is usually the goal of replacement - not taking hormone levels to that of a 20-year old! If your symptoms have been alleviated, and it is clear that your hormone levels have been raised to a reasonable level for your age, this ought to be sufficient. Therefore, the optimal ranges for a post-menopausal woman provided in this chapter are merely a guideline. You may achieve symptom relief with lower levels than these.

I have already mentioned that almost all women require progesterone replacement post-menopause, as the loss of progesterone is so dramatic. Even though both progesterone and oestradiol levels have fallen, oestrogen dominance is usually worsened since the progesterone level has fallen so much.

### How sex hormone replacement is taken in non-cycling/post-menopausal women

The adrenals know nothing of cycles and make their small level of progesterone and tiny amount of testosterone every day of the month. More testosterone and some oestradiol is produced in the peripheral tissues through conversion of other hormones like DHEA.

Getting low levels of sex hormones back to reasonable post-menopausal levels will help to maintain good health and well-being. Any supplementation would need to be done on every day of the month to mimic post-menopausal production.

So, non-cycling/post-menopausal women use any needed progesterone or oestradiol on every day of the month. A 2-3 day break every month or two, or a 1 day break per week, help to keep the sex hormone receptors sensitive.

### Delivery options for sex hormone replacement in non-cycling/post-menopausal women

There are many forms of sex hormone replacement these days. Delivery can be through bio-identical transdermal creams & oils, buccal lozenges (they attach to the gums and absorb sublingually), or oral bio-identical capsules. There is a long history of using vaginal delivery for hormone treatment. It is thought that this most closely mimics natural delivery to the target tissues. However, some products, and some delivery methods, work for some women and not for others. For instance, some women find that bio-identical transdermal creams work well, but for others they simply do not raise hormone levels at all. This may be more apparent with progesterone cream, as it contains a much higher volume of the actual hormone compared to oestradiol or testosterone creams, i.e. there is far more hormone to absorb through the skin.

Do your own research. There is nearly always a product that works, if this is the choice that you wish to make.

### Safety - there are some critical things to be aware of

*Firstly, for those post-menopausal women who have a uterus, the use of any oestrogen replacement must be accompanied by sufficient progesterone to remove any uterine cancer risk.*

*Secondly*, many women find taking progesterone near bedtime helps them sleep better. Whereas, oestradiol is usually taken in the morning, as it can sometimes be too stimulatory when taken in the evening. The question sometimes comes up as to whether the progesterone is still giving protection against uterine cancer during the following day. The answer is yes. Progesterone, especially via capsules, tends to stay pretty steady in the bloodstream. Significantly, elevated levels are typically seen in the 8-12 hour range after taking the progesterone. However, you do not get back to baseline until 24-hours or more. So, taking progesterone, even at bedtime, provides good cover over the next full day. This is especially true if the oestradiol being used is oral, as this takes time for it to even get to the target tissues.

*Thirdly, in the case of progesterone replacement, it has been shown that synthetic progesterone (progestogen/progestin) is linked to higher risk of breast cancer. Ideally, both natural (bio-identical) oestradiol and progesterone will be used.* However, the French have a safe history of using oral natural progesterone capsules combined with synthetic oestradiol (normal oestrogen HRT). *The combination of bio-identical progesterone combined with synthetic oestradiol has been shown to be very safe compared to conventional HRT (which uses synthetic oestradiol and progestogen).* See *reference 2* in Resources at the end of the chapter on the use of synthetic oestrogen accompanied by natural progesterone.

### A few notes on sex hormone replacement in non-cycling/post-menopausal women

Oestrogen increases the protein that *binds* thyroid hormone. This happens when oestrogen levels increase, regardless of the type of oestrogen used. This can cause hypothyroid symptoms and possibly a need for an increase in thyroid medication.

Because of this, oral oestrogen should usually be taken at a different time to thyroid medication. Some sources indicate an hour apart is fine, others recommend four hours (timing is not a concern with creams, gels, or other non-oral types.). The best way to tell if your thyroid dosage needs to be increased, or your oestrogen needs to be timed differently, is to monitor symptoms and signs after starting oestrogen.

Oestrogen is typically used once per day, in the mornings, as it can be energizing. However, this is very individual so patients may find other times work better for them. Sometimes, oestrogen is dosed multiple times daily.

Progesterone is typically dosed just before bed because it can sometimes cause sleepiness. This effect tends to be more common for people with normal or low night-time cortisol levels. This is particularly true for oral progesterone, as this form tends to increase the metabolites that cause drowsiness.

For people with high cortisol at night, using progesterone at that time can make issues like insomnia worse. Patients who have higher night-time cortisol levels, or who experience high cortisol symptoms after starting progesterone, may want to consider changing their dosing to morning or afternoon or splitting their dose to see if these symptoms resolve. Some women do have success when progesterone is dosed morning and at bedtime. Some experimentation may be necessary with timing.

If testosterone is being replaced, it is sometimes dosed once per day in the morning or less frequently, such as every other day or twice weekly. Again this is individual and depends on the symptoms experienced by the patient.

Anecdotally, I have been told that some women find that their cortisol becomes too high if they use progesterone supplementation. This is puzzling, as progesterone tends to counter cortisol-effect within the cells. We also know from research that extra progesterone will not be shunted into cortisol, if there is no HP dysfunction. Hence, I can only find one reason to explain this. As mentioned in Chapter 11, any transdermal progesterone use has the potential to corrupt a cortisol saliva test result, depending on the lab assay method being used. The molecular structure of progesterone is close enough to cortisol to do this, whereas oestrogen and testosterone, for example, are not. But this is just speculation on my part.

Usually high cortisol produces the symptoms I describe in Chapter 5, including high blood pressure, facial flushing, fluid retention, insomnia etc. If progesterone addition always acted to boost cortisol, every woman who is cycling would have higher cortisol in the second half of her cycle! Clearly, this is not true, so some other more subtle explanation is required. I am just speculating above about possible explanations. It is an outstanding question mark as I complete the book.

## RESOLVING ANY SEX HORMONE ISSUE CAN BE CRITICAL

It should be obvious from this chapter that, if there is a sex hormone issue, it can seriously affect your health and well-being. There are complex interactions with all the hormones within the tissues and at the HP level. Thyroid treatment may be more difficult to manage when a myriad of other issues are also present.

If there is a sex hormone issue detected through testing, there may be multiple ways to resolve it. Some form of intervention may well be required if you are to really feel well and to protect your long-term health.

Please seek professional help with an experienced specialist to assess and potentially correct any sex hormone issues. Progesterone and oestradiol are very important to manage at healthy levels. If your specialist is willing to treat with testosterone (if required) this is so much the better.

## MEN AND TESTOSTERONE

In the case of men, the symptoms of low testosterone can certainly cause problems that may complicate thyroid hormone treatment. Low testosterone has been linked to many health issues in men including cardiovascular disease, high blood pressure and obesity, and the more obvious loss of muscle strength, low energy/drive, depression, low libido and erectile dysfunction. ***Men require optimal, not just in-range testosterone levels for well-being and long-term health.***

Fortunately, low testosterone is very easy to test for these days. It may well be worth testing for total testosterone, free testosterone, Sex Hormone Binding Globulin (SHBG which binds some of the total testosterone and stops it from being bio-available). Your doctor can use these results to assess the complete situation.

These are all ***blood test results***, as they are still regarded as the most accurate way to test male sex hormones. The ranges presented are for adult males in the 20-50 year old range. For some reason, the male sex hormone values vary significantly by country, region and lab, so these are just a guideline. You will need to work with your own doctor to assess the health of your sex hormones.

***Testosterone is ideally tested in the morning within 2 hours of awakening, when testosterone is at its highest.***

### Total Testosterone ranges

| | |
|---|---|
| US units: | 240-1100 ng/dL |
| European units: | 8.4-32 nmol/L |
| Optimal: | 800-1100 ng/dL = 26-32 nmol/L |

While testosterone levels naturally decrease with age, low testosterone in men may result in a number of symptoms including low sex drive, difficulty achieving erections, low semen volume, hair loss, fatigue and lack of energy, loss of muscle mass, increase in body fat, decrease in bone mass, and mood changes. The goal of testosterone restoration, in most cases, is to restore youthful blood levels of the hormone.

According to some sources, an **optimal level for all men would be in the upper third of the reference range** for men aged 21 to 49 years, and that any supplementation should aim to restore hormone levels to that range.

### Free Testosterone ranges

| | |
|---|---|
| US units: | 4-20 ng/dL |
| European units: | 0.25-0.7 nmol/L |
| Optimal: | Top quartile of the reference range, |
| | e.g. if 4-20 ngl/dL was the range then 16-20 ngl/dL is the top quartile. |

Note: **the above are just examples of ranges**. This test in particular, may have ranges that vary considerably by lab. The free testosterone test is a difficult lab test to run, so this probably explains the variation in the ranges. Endocrinologists usually only accept that someone has low free testosterone if the result falls in the bottom 2.5% of the reference range or below, i.e. there are 97.5% of other people with levels higher than you!

Free testosterone is the unbound form that is biologically available to cell receptor sites throughout the body. Measuring free testosterone blood levels is the most accurate way of assessing testosterone status in men. **Like total testosterone, it needs to be tested in the morning within 2 hours of awakening, when testosterone is at its highest**.

If you have results for total testosterone, albumin and SHBG, an estimate of free testosterone may be made. Here is a free testosterone calculator: http://www.issam.ch/freetesto.htm

### Sex hormone Binding Globulin (SHBG) ranges

| | |
|---|---|
| US units: | 10-57 nmol/L |
| European units: | 13-71 nmol/L |
| Optimal: | <50 nmol/L |

SHBG binds with testosterone and other androgens, so in men, we do not want to see high levels of SHBG. If SHBG is particularly low, it is likely that thyroid hormone is low, or that sex hormones are low.

Note: the use of stinging nettle root 250-500mg 2x per day can, in some cases, help to lower SHBG and free up more testosterone.

### *Free Androgen Index (FAI)*

FAI = (total testosterone divided by SHBG) x 100%

SHBG and total testosterone need to be in the same units before calculating this.

FAI is useful as a tool during treatment to see which direction things are going in, i.e. with improvement, the FAI ought to be rising. It is no replacement for testing, or estimating free testosterone.

## Treatment options

Low testosterone is usually easy to treat and there are multiple delivery mechanisms, e.g. transdermal gels, patches, injections and implants.

If low testosterone or low free testosterone levels are present, this may be impacting thyroid hormone treatment, or at least may confuse the symptomatic picture because some of the symptoms may be similar, e.g. lethargy, weakness, depression.

## NOTES ON PROLACTIN FOR WOMEN AND MEN

This is unlikely to apply to you. However, in a very few people, this information may be relevant. I am including it in order to be complete.

Prolactin is a hormone produced by the pituitary gland, which is involved in the production and control of adrenal, thyroid and sex hormones. Prolactin is mostly known for controlling a woman's breast milk during pregnancy and nursing. Some medications can elevate prolactin, as can kidney failure or chest trauma. However, when prolactin is elevated in either women or men, and none of the above applies, this can indicate the presence of a (typically) benign pituitary tumour known as a prolactinoma.

If prolactinomas in women are small, they may not produce many symptoms. If they are larger and produce high levels of prolactin, this can cause absent or irregular periods (interfering with the production of progesterone), infertility, low levels of other sex hormones (particularly estrogen), low sex drive, and/or a milky breast discharge in the absence of pregnancy.

In men, even smaller tumours, causing slight elevations in prolactin, can lead to painful and awkward symptoms including headaches or vision problems (if the tumour is pressing on the nerves behind the eyes), or low libido, infertility, and erectile dysfunction due to the lowering effect of prolactin on the production of testosterone.

Prolactinoma tumours are typically diagnosed first by blood tests for prolactin, often multiple times, spaced a week or two apart. These tests should always be taken within 3 hours of waking, as prolactin levels vary throughout the day. If prolactin is consistently elevated, a pituitary MRI will often be performed to confirm the size and placement of the prolactinoma.

Typically, prolactinomas are treated using a medication that is taken orally, once or twice weekly. Depending on the size of the tumour, the medication is taken for several years for smaller tumours. For larger tumours the medication may need to be taken indefinitely. Tumour regrowth often reoccurs, so prolactin levels and tumour size are monitored carefully.

If either women or men test prolactin and it is consistently elevated, please seek a specialist. Prolactinomas, while noncancerous, can cause cascading impacts to adrenal, thyroid, and sex hormone function, in addition to the symptoms above.

Note: a common cause of mildly elevated prolactin is hypothyroidism.

### Final comments on sex hormones

The above provides some *guidelines* for anyone who suspects that their sex hormones are a problem. It is a starting point and may be useful when working with a specialist. If you can find a doctor who focuses on sex hormones, this is advisable. It is a complex area and there are many different ways of addressing issues. If someone requires sex hormone supplementation, finding the right type of medication and the right means of taking it, are critical. Having a highly competent doctor supporting you is extremely important.

### RESOURCES

Here are a few useful references:

1. *Steroidogenesis diagram -*
https://upload.wikimedia.org/wikipedia/commons/thumb/1/13/Steroidogenesis.svg/865px-Steroidogenesis.svg.png (shows the pathways involved in the production of cortisol, aldosterone and sex hormones).

2. *Progestins and progesterone in hormone replacement therapy and the risk of breast cancer -* Campagnoli, Clavel-Chapelon, Kaaks, Peris and Berrino -
See: https://www.ncbi.nlm.nih.gov/pmc/articles/PMC1974841/
(very interesting study in France that shows that breast cancer risk is linked to the use of synthetic progesterone/progestins/progestogen).

3. *What Your Doctor May Not Tell You About Menopause -* John R. Lee, M.D.

4. *Testosterone for Life -* Abraham Morgentaler, M.D.

5. *Can LDL cholesterol be too low? Possible risks of extremely low levels -* Olsson AG, Angelin B, Assmann G, Binder CJ, Björkhem I, Cedazo-Minguez A, Cohen J, von Eckardstein A, Farinaro E, Müller-Wieland D, Parhofer KG, Parini P, Rosenson RS, Starup-Linde J[13], Tikkanen MJ, Yvan-Charvet L.
J Intern Med. 2017 Jun;281(6):534-553. doi: 10.1111/joim.12614.
See: https://www.ncbi.nlm.nih.gov/pubmed/28295777 for the abstract and
https://onlinelibrary.wiley.com/doi/pdf/10.1111/joim.12614 for the full article

# Chapter 22

# Less Common Issues to Investigate, Test & Deal With

Many other problems can interfere with or totally derail thyroid hormone treatment. It would be impossible to ask someone to have all these ruled out prior to starting treatment. However, once in thyroid treatment, if it is not going smoothly, and there are no other obvious reasons, this chapter may provide you with ideas for further investigations.

Each short section in this chapter will say a little about the possible problem, and how it might affect thyroid treatment. You will have to do your own research, if you think the topic could be relevant. There are books, Internet sites and Internet patient forums on most of these topics, as well as doctors who are experienced in them.

I will just take each topic one at a time. There is no priority order to this.

## GUT HEALTH

Apart from pain, discomfort, bloating and obvious issues like this, why might a thyroid patient under treatment suspect a gut health issue? The thyroid patient ought to have tested vitamin B12, folate, vitamin D and iron. If more than one nutrient was low, a gut issue might already be suspected. Moreover, if thyroid hormone dosage is increased, and a full thyroid panel shows no noticeable changes in TSH, FT4 or FT3, I might be concerned that the thyroid medication is not being absorbed properly.

Absorption issues in the gut can be caused by a gut permeability problem. This is sometimes referred to as leaky gut. Gut permeability issues can quite frequently be caused by systemic candida. Candida can itself be induced by hypothyroidism. If absorption issues are suspected, a knowledgeable physician should investigate them.

Absorption issues in the gut can affect a wider range of vitamins including vitamin A, B vitamins, vitamin K and trace minerals. Of course it could affect your thyroid medication itself, and any other medication that you take orally.

Sometimes low stomach acid can contribute to absorption problems.

If you, or your doctor, begin to suspect absorption or gut health issues, your doctor needs to run a wider range of tests to begin to investigate this. These will almost certainly include a complete blood count, liver & kidney function tests, electrolytes, and tests for inflammation: C-reactive protein (CRP), plasma viscosity (PV) and erythrocyte sedimentation rate (ESR). He may wish to run other tests depending on your symptoms and medical history.

I do not think you should guess, or try to work out the cause yourself. The consequences of malabsorption are so profound that this needs to be investigated thoroughly by a competent doctor.

You may wish to consider dietary adjustments if you have enough symptoms to suggest gut permeability issues.

The health of the gut is critical. It is the foundation that allows raw materials to reach our energy system.

## BLOOD SUGAR CONTROL

If blood sugar fluctuates considerably, remains low or rises too high, this will dramatically effect how you feel. You now know enough about our energy system to realise that the mitochondria require a flow of glucose. Without this flow, our energy system slows down. The foundation of this requires a healthy dietary intake, good gut health and absorption of food, and healthy adrenal function (cortisol needs to maintain blood sugar levels). We also need correct insulin levels (and no insulin resistance), for the blood sugar level to be controlled, and to allow the transport of glucose past the cell membranes to the mitochondria. To be honest we are so complex that I am surprised that so many of us work as well as we actually do!

Clearly, diet plays a huge part in all of this. Extremely low carb or low calorie diets are not a good idea. Skipping meals is also not a smart move.

If you have hypocortisolism, then, as you know by now, low blood sugar is likely to result.

Some investigations might need to be done if you or your doctor suspects blood sugar issues. The main tests for measuring the amount of glucose in the blood are:

- A random blood glucose test.
- Fasting blood glucose test.
- The HbA1c blood test - gives an overall idea of average blood sugar levels.
- Oral glucose tolerance test - a more complex test that shows what happens after you digest glucose. It can expose fluctuations in blood sugar and can be useful.
- Home blood sugar monitoring - can be helpful to carry out some investigations at home.
- Urine test for glucose.

If you suspect blood sugar issues, talk to your doctor. If the issues are significant and remain undetected, it can make understanding, and correcting problems during thyroid treatment very difficult.

## ZINC/COPPER BALANCE

It is reasonably common for those with thyroid conditions to have a copper imbalance. This can affect the way thyroid hormones work. It can also lead to other issues like migraines, allergies and depression. High copper can elevate oestrogen in women. A copper/zinc imbalance can also cause ferritin to remain low, even though the other iron labs look fine.

In hypothyroidism, the issue is usually high copper (copper toxicity). However, it can occasionally be low copper. In either case, if thyroid treatment is not going well, this is an issue for you to consider looking into.

What are the main causes of copper toxicity?

- Water supplies containing high copper levels - so drinking filtered tap water is a good idea.
- Copper plumbing within our homes - this can lead to us absorbing copper through drinking water and even when showering.
- Intra-uterine devices with copper - are likely to raise copper levels in women using them.
- Adrenal issues can lead to high copper - healthy adrenal function produces a copper-binding protein. When there is some type of adrenal issue, they produce less of this and copper levels can build up.
- Low zinc - zinc is necessary to balance the levels of copper, and so a zinc deficiency can lead to excess copper levels.

Testing for an unbound copper issue will require **blood tests of: serum copper, serum zinc and ceruloplasmin.**

Some practitioners have faith in a hair mineral analysis test, as it is relatively inexpensive and shows a range of minerals that might be high or low. However, I understand that the blood tests I have just mentioned provide the most accurate method of checking the unbound (bio-available) copper level and any zinc/copper imbalance.

Here is a simple formula to get a rough picture of your free copper levels:

- Free copper % = (total serum copper in ug/dl) - (ceruloplasmin in mg/dL x 3).
- Note: ug/dL is sometimes written as mcg/dL.
- The healthy range for free copper % is 5-15%.

To assess zinc/copper ratio:

- You first have to put copper and zinc into the same units (use an on-line conversion tool).
- Then just divide the serum zinc by the serum copper level (when in the same units).
- The zinc/copper ratio should be 1.2-1.4 : 1.
- If zinc/copper is less than 1, your zinc is low compared to copper, which is undesirable.
- Zinc is best in the top third of the range.

If you think you have a zinc/copper issue, or wish to exclude it, you could choose to get the tests done. Then take your results to a competent physician who knows how to interpret them, and who can provide advice to correct any imbalance if necessary. There are also Internet based groups on Facebook that focus on this type of issue.

## INFECTIONS (e.g. Lyme Disease, Root Canal, Sinus, Epstein Barr/Glandular Fever etc.)

All infections can cause issues with thyroid treatment and some are worse than others. Infections drag the immune system down and tend to lower cortisol through adrenal stress.

Lyme disease is one of the most insidious of infections. It can occur when a tick infected with Borrelia virus bites someone. Symptoms of Lyme disease can include an initial rash, general un-wellness, unexplained flu-like symptoms, aches, light or noise sensitivity, brain fog, fatigue, a stiff neck, numbness or tingling. The infection can spread to anywhere in the body. As a result, people can develop issues with their endocrine and neurological systems etc. It should be obvious that if someone contracts Lyme disease, it might simply appear to be another set of symptoms of hypothyroidism. Conversely, Lyme disease could cause the onset of thyroid hormone issues. In any event, it can make treatment with thyroid hormones incredibly difficult due to hypocortisolism and sensitivity to thyroid hormone.

I have experience of thyroid patients with root canal, sinus and other infections that have had hypocortisolism issues or cortisol rhythm issues as a result. These, too, can make treatment with thyroid hormones extremely difficult. Trying to reach a therapeutic dosage with any of the thyroid treatments may be next to impossible in the presence of these infections.

So, if you know that you have some kind of infection, it is really important to get this properly treated.

If thyroid treatment has not been going well and the more obvious issues have been excluded, ask your doctor to check for the possibility of an infection.

## TOXICITY (INCLUDING ENVIRONMENTAL TOXINS)

Let me just illustrate one example of how toxicity can cause issues. It is known that some toxins can compromise liver function. Those with liver function issues can have high sensitivity to thyroid hormone treatments, especially those that have T3 in them. This can cause high heart rate during treatment, amongst other things, making it hard to get to the correct thyroid hormone dosage.

Unfortunately, there are many chemicals in our environment that are toxic. Some of these can be avoided, whereas others are getting harder to avoid as they are in our water supply, the air that we breathe, and our foods.

*Pesticides* are used in the production of our food. Livestock are often given antibiotics and treated with pesticides. The foods that livestock are fed have often been treated at some stage with pesticides.

*Mercury* is highly toxic and is found in amalgam based dental fillings. It is also used in the composition of some vaccines. Mercury stays in the body for a long time, and can affect the biochemical pathways associated with thyroid hormones. Many people opt for non-amalgam based fillings these days, or have their existing amalgam fillings removed and swapped for composite ones. Mercury fillings should only be removed by a dentist who has been trained in their safe removal. Otherwise, mercury can be ingested into the body. See **reference 1** in Resources at the end of the chapter.

*Heavy Metals* like lead, cadmium and mercury are produced by some industries and contaminate the food chain (fish especially). They are all capable of blocking the uptake of selenium, crucial in the processing of thyroid hormones. Cadmium is also known to induce a lowering of TSH.

*Dioxins and PCBs (polychlorinated biphenols)* if ingested, these remain in fatty tissues in our bodies for many years. Dioxins interfere with the uptake of iodine and how it is processed into thyroid hormones. PCBs are used in many electrical products, in plastic manufacture, paints, adhesives, flame-retardants and inks. There has been a phasing out of their use, but the contamination of the environment and food chain has already occurred. Dioxins and PCBs are toxic and can damage our immune systems, liver and the processing of thyroid hormones. PCBs can also prevent enough thyroid hormone from binding to a protein called transthyretin, which is the protein responsible for carrying thyroid hormone to the brain. PCBs and other chemical contaminants can directly reduce thyroid hormone production of T4 and T3 and speed up thyroid hormone clearance.

*Fluorides* are compounds containing fluorine, and they are all toxic to the body to some extent. Fluoride tends to destroy and disrupt enzymes and can have a disastrous effect on the processing of thyroid hormones. A common exposure to fluoride is from toothpaste, although we have the option to buy toothpaste without fluoride. Fluorides are present in many other applications, including numerous drugs like antibiotics and anaesthetics. Fluoride is also added to the water supply in some areas to reduce tooth decay. Buying bottled water or using a home water filter system can remove fluoride and other contaminants. I am a believer in home water filtering technology. It can take out contaminants like fluoride, xenoestrogens etc.

*Silica, Beryllium, Aluminium and Fluorine* are all capable of increasing the level of protein Gq/11 which can reduce the action of the T3 thyroid hormone within our cells. The Gq/11 protein also desensitizes the thyroid to the stimulation of TSH, which in turn, will lower the production of T4 and T3 from the thyroid.

Some toxins like the heavy metals may show up in mineral tests. If you continue to have thyroid treatment issues, this is another area that could be investigated.

## HYPOTHALAMUS / PITUITARY ISSUES

There are several reasons why hypothalamus or pituitary issues might be considered to be a possibility.

If during thyroid treatment your cortisol remains low, hypothalamic-pituitary (HP) dysfunction might be suspected. Morning blood cortisol might be low, a cortisol saliva test might show low free cortisol across the day, but you might respond well to a synacthen test

(ACTH Stim. test). Note: I am assuming that you have already tested cortisol before treatment, and if it was severely low, you will have been seen and investigated by an endocrinologist or specialist.

TSH may have been low during the diagnosis stage when a full thyroid panel was run, but if FT4 and FT3 were also low, this would be an odd situation.

If hypothalamic-pituitary dysfunction were being considered, your endocrinologist or doctor might test the full range of pituitary hormones: ACTH, FSH, LH, GH, PRL and TSH. Sometimes only some of these are low.

If hypocortisolism is thought to be due to a possible HP dysfunction, your doctor might arrange for a hospital based insulin tolerance test (see Chapter 11).

If your doctor is concerned about possible pituitary or hypothalamus involvement, this needs to get ruled out, as it may be impossible to resolve symptoms without a proper diagnosis. Some intervention may be needed in order to correct any other low hormones that are being caused by the hypothalamic-pituitary dysfunction.

However, most commonly occurring HP-dysfunction is not dramatic, and it is of unknown origin, making it hard to diagnose with a specific test.

## MITOCHONDRIAL PROBLEMS

In Chapters 2 and 6, I explained the vital importance of the mitochondria within our energy system. I direct you to Dr Sarah Myhill's excellent book on the subject for further information.

Proper diagnosis of mitochondrial issues is a specialist area. If you or your doctor suspect this could be a problem, locating a specialist would be necessary. Dr. Myhill's book describes a programme for rehabilitating the mitochondria with nutritional supplements (see the Resources at the end of Chapter 6).

## GENETIC DEFECTS

The DIO1 and DIO2 gene defects can impact T4 to T3 conversion in individuals with these polymorphisms. Since the D2 deiodinase enzyme is far more effective in converting T4 to T3 than D1, the DIO2 mutation is more important to test for. I know of patients who have had their T3 medication restored on prescription, when they proved that they had the DIO2 defect. *Regenerus Labs* provides testing for DIO2. Other companies offer people a full work up of their genetic information, but not all may include DIO1 and DIO2; so, you will need to check with them first. If you get a full genome analysis other faulty genes may be revealed, including some of the ones relevant to MTHFR.

If you have one of the DIO1 or DIO2 gene defects, you begin to have conversion issues. If you inherit one of these mutations from one parent it will reduce ability to convert T4 to T3. However, the issue gets worse if you inherit a mutation from *both parents*, e.g. having two copies of DIO1 is worse than one copy. These can affect you in many ways. It can lower T3 levels and induce hypothyroidism. It can even cause hypocortisolism, as the pituitary uses D2 to maintain its extremely high levels of T3. As we get older we are more likely to be subject to poor conversion if we have one or both of these mutations. In my case, I believe my DIO1 and DIO2 gene defects became a problem some time during my twenties. The defects were not causing symptoms before then; it is thought that the body can compensate in young people. As For me personally, I believe it was a factor in both hypothyroidism and hypocortisolism.

I do believe that all thyroid patients should be aware of the presence of DIO1 and DIO2 genetic defects. They can significantly affect the conversion of T4 to T3, and guide you as to the most appropriate choice of thyroid medication treatment, i.e. if you have either of them; it is far more likely that you will need thyroid medication containing at least some T3.

There may be many other gene defects that could adversely affect other processes within your body. In some cases, other impaired bio-chemical processes can make it more difficult to recover from hypothyroidism.

You may wish to investigate this area yourself.

## MTHFR

MTHFR stands for methylene-tetrahydrofolate reductase. It is an enzyme involved in the conversion of folate that you ingest, into the active form (5-methyltetrahydrofolate).

I explained in Chapter 10 that folate deficiency can appear like a B12 deficiency, i.e. with symptoms that overlap with thyroid symptoms. Consequently, a MTHFR problem can confuse your thyroid hormone treatment.

Why is folate important in our bodies?

- Folate is critical in the synthesis of DNA, RNA and SAMe - all needed for cellular health.
- Various crucial reactions in the body require the donation of methyl groups to become active - so these need folate.
- Amino acid metabolism requires folate. Amino acid metabolism is important for our neurotransmitters and detoxification.
- Red and white blood cell and platelet production also requires folate.
- Folate is critical for the detox of homocysteine.

None of the above happens efficiently if folate cannot be converted to its active form. For that, the MTHFR enzyme needs to be present and doing its job.

The proper conversion of folate to the active form allows the production of various methyl groups in the body. These groups have different and critical functions in the body. If you do not have enough methyl groups, you will not be able to use the vitamins and minerals that you eat or supplement with.

If someone has problems with a gene that affects the MTHFR enzyme, they may have to use different forms of supplementation to provide the active forms of various vitamins, e.g. methyl-cobalamin (active B12), methyl-folate (active folate). In the supplementation regime I suggested in Chapter 12, I have proposed the active forms already.

MTHFR and other types of SNP (single nucleotide polymorphism) may exist. These can be detected with genetic screening. There are usually ways of working around any problems. See the previous section on Genetic Defects for the approach to testing and assessment. As I mentioned in the previous section on genetic defects, issues like MTHFR can get in the way of a full recovery from hypothyroidism.

There are Internet groups where patients with this issue can give support to each other.

So, this is yet another area that you could look into if thyroid hormone treatment is not going so well. See *reference 2* in Resources.

## PYROLURIA

Pyroluria is a genetic issue that involves an abnormality in the manufacture of haemoglobin, the protein that holds iron inside our red blood cells. People with this disorder produce too much of a bi-product of haemoglobin manufacture called Kryptopyrrole (KP). KP binds to vitamin B6 and zinc and makes them unavailable in the body, which is obviously highly undesirable. These essential nutrients are then removed from the bloodstream and excreted into the urine. Hence, pyroluria is detected by the chemical analysis of urine.

The effect of pyroluria can be varied depending on the severity.

Most individuals with pyroluria have symptoms of zinc or B6 deficiencies. These include poor stress control, nervousness, anxiety, mood swings, inner tension, irritability, short-term memory issues and depression. They also cannot make enough serotonin (vitamin B6 is needed to make it). Patients with pyroluria are stress intolerant. They seem to be especially vulnerable to cumulative stress over many days.

Pyroluria is treated by restoring vitamin B6 and zinc. The type of replacement used is critical, and expert help needs to be sought to get the right type/level of treatment. Other nutrients may also be needed. Again, it is best to get expert help with this.

So, a patient with hypothyroidism may not get full symptom relief if they have any form of pyroluria. Hence, pyroluria can confuse the diagnosis of hypothyroidism and vice versa.

## ELECTROLYTE IMBALANCE

Electrolytes are minerals that contain an electric charge. The sodium and potassium electrolytes in our bloodstream are critical in the function of muscles, nerves and neurons (brain cells).

The adrenals are key to regulating the balance of electrolytes in the body. Consequently, an electrolyte imbalance can result from adrenal issues.

Getting an electrolyte test done is fairly easy, as it is one of the most standard tests that your doctor could run.

In the early stages of adrenal stress it is common to see high cortisol accompanied by high sodium. Low potassium impacts thyroid hormone activity at the cellular level.

I would consider getting the electrolytes tested if problems persist. If there is some kind of imbalance, discuss this with your doctor. There may also be some helpful suggestions amongst patient groups.

## ANTI-DEPRESSANT USE & NEUROTRANSMITTER DISTURBANCES

If the neurotransmitters (e.g. dopamine, serotonin) get out of balance or low, this may affect the smoothness of any thyroid treatment.

Over the years, I have witnessed individuals with hypothyroidism and hypocortisolism that proved resistant to improvement. A number of these patients had been on anti-depressants for some time. Those taking anti-anxiety drugs (not strictly anti-depressants) like those in the benzodiazepine family were struggling more than most. Gaining tolerance to a therapeutic dose of thyroid hormone was extraordinarily difficult for these people, even for several months or years after ceasing to take the anti-depressant/anti-anxiety medication.

Neurotransmitter changes/disturbances can be significant in adrenal and thyroid issues. I cannot say I understand the mechanisms at work with anti-depressant or anti-anxiety medications, but they have been observed to cause problems during thyroid treatment, especially when hypocortisolism has been present.

Anti-depressant use can also have unwanted side effects, including reducing melatonin production, and depleting vitamins and minerals. A patient who is taking an anti-depressant should consider ensuring they are on a sound nutritional support regime because there is the potential for lower than normal vitamins and minerals (see Chapter 12).

It is extremely dangerous to just stop anti-depressant or anti-anxiety medication use. I am not arguing for that. I am just trying to make people aware that there may be potential problems. Any adjustment in a patient's medication must be done with their doctor's full involvement and approval.

## OTHER VITAMINS / MINERALS

There are other possible vitamin and mineral deficiencies that might be relevant to you if treatment is not progressing well. Vitamin A is needed to produce TSH and to convert T4 to T3. Note: vitamin A is best absorbed when ingested with some protein. It is essential not to over-dose on vitamin A, so this needs to have been tested, found low and an appropriate treatment put in place by your doctor.

Magnesium is required in many processes in the body and is extremely low in many people. Magnesium is used along with selenium and zinc in the conversion of T4 to T3. Many of us are low in magnesium, and it is very safe to supplement with it to tolerance (some forms can cause diarrhoea, so I prefer the glycinate or biglycinate versions).

Note: magnesium, selenium and zinc are all in my basic supplementation regime.

## OTHER DISEASES

This is a catchall category at the end of this chapter.

It is possible for a patient to have struggled for a long time to recover from hypothyroidism. They may have tried all the treatments, even as far as T3-Only. They may have been working on correcting any hypocortisolism. Any nutritional supplement issues may have been addressed. Yet, there may still be issues.

In a few, unlucky cases, there may have been something else going on all the time behind the scenes.

It is disheartening for these people and for all those who may have been trying to support them in their huge effort for symptom relief.

I have worked with thousands of thyroid patients over the past 10 years, and occasionally something like this happens.

In one case, someone that I had tried really hard to help finally got a diagnosis of Mast Cell Disease (Mastocytosis). Mast cells produce histamine and other chemicals that trigger allergic reactions. There are many symptoms associated with this. It produces a huge strain on the adrenals and makes raising cortisol extremely difficult. Thus successful thyroid treatment is hard to achieve when something undiagnosed like this is happening.

Now that she has a diagnosis, I hope that the lady concerned can also resolve her thyroid and adrenal issues (even if she needs intervention with HC to achieve this).

## CONCLUSIONS

The above represent some of the conditions and factors that may need to be considered, if thyroid hormone treatment continues to be problematic.

The biggest challenge may be in recognising that one or more of these, or other issues, are present. I hope the information in this chapter at least provides some food for thought, if thyroid treatment has reached some kind of impasse.

## RESOURCES

Here are a few useful references:

1. ***It's All in Your Head: The link Between Mercury Amalgams and Illness*** - Hal A. Huggins
2. ***MTHFR Basics*** - Benjamin Lynch

# Chapter 23

## Gain Some Control, Do it Early & Do Not Accept Roadblocks

I have been living with thyroid hormone concerns, and thyroid hormone treatment, since I was about 28 years old. I am 60 this year.

The only way that I could get well was through the use of T3-Only, and by inventing a good protocol for its safe and effective use, including the creation of CT3M.

If I had listened to my doctors and endocrinologists early in my illness, I would probably be dead by now. On T4-Only, I was virtually bed bound in the first 7 years of my illness and used to pass out regularly due to low blood pressure. Different doctors and endocrinologists offered me various diagnoses. I was told that I had chronic fatigue syndrome (CFS), myalgic encephalitis (ME), depression, and 'something else going on', i.e. anything but an incorrectly treated thyroid hormone disorder. My very low free cortisol and total cortisol, detected from a 24-hour urinary cortisol test, was ignored. I had passed a Synacthen test, so there was no Addison's disease, even though my daily cortisol levels were low enough to cause serious symptoms.

Eventually, I realised that I had to gain some control of my health, if I was to get well. I could no longer leave my health in the hands of others. After that, even when I told doctors that I felt well on T3-Only, I was informed that my previous blood test results were normal on T4-Only, so I should return to using that treatment! I had years and years of poor medical care. I lost a great deal that was important to me in the process.

It became obvious to me that I had to gain some control of my health and argue for what I needed.

I did this when there were no books on using thyroid hormones, no **Recovering with T3** book, and no Internet, hence no forums from which to seek support. It was hard, and it has had huge costs for me personally.

If someone gets a diagnosis of a thyroid hormone disorder and is given T4-Only/Levo/Synthroid and gets well, this is wonderful, and I say good luck to them! However, for many, it is a vast struggle, and it can take a very long time for them to get well again.

There are so many reasons why T4-Only will not ever work for some thyroid patients. I have outlined many of the reasons in this book; a defective DIO1 or DIO2 gene, loss of thyroid tissue through thyroidectomy or Hashimoto's (loss of T4 to T3 conversion), low ferritin, low vitamin D and hypocortisolism are just a few. Sometimes, someone has to move to another treatment in order to get well.

This book is a tool. It is a manual. It is perhaps a combat manual, because often you have to recover your health. You can use it to understand your own energy system. You can use it to understand which tests are important, as well as their limitations. You can use it to work through the process of getting well again. This manual is written to help you on your own journey, from suspicions of possible hypothyroidism, right through to recovery. It may not contain every single piece of information that all of you need in order to get well. It will not replace working with a good doctor. However, it has a lot of straightforward, practical advice and it is consistent with up to date research at this time. Take from it what is useful to you.

In order to get well, it is sometimes necessary for a patient to take a far greater interest in their condition than with other health issues. If someone does not take a keen interest, there is a risk that they may not get correctly diagnosed or treated.

Many thyroid patients come up against the situation where symptoms are still present, but their doctor tells them that they are correctly treated because their thyroid labs are in range! Be prepared for this beforehand, and use as many of the arguments in this book as necessary for either further increases in medication, or a change in the medication type. Use some of the research references if you think they will help. If you have to, be prepared to find a new doctor!

Please try to get the right tests and treatment. Be prepared to work even harder to find a supportive physician, as this can make **all** the difference. It is so much easier to work with a good, competent and empathetic doctor. Even in this circumstance, please keep an interest in your treatment and be a full participant in all discussions regarding it. You own your body - no one else does!

**You may have to convince your doctor to treat you correctly**

You may be faced with a situation where your doctor is not treating your hypothyroidism correctly. Changing doctor may work. However, it would be easier if you could convince your doctor to change their mind.

Your TSH may be normal but you can still be hypothyroid. If you want to obtain the right treatment from your current doctor, you may need to convince them that you need T3 in addition to T4 in some ratio (or NDT). You will also need to convince your doctor that the TSH cannot be used to guide the treatment, whether it was high or normal to start with.

Without the ability to confidently argue for these points, you may struggle to persuade your doctor away from the old and incorrect ways. Worse case, you may even succumb to your doctor's perceived expertise and do what you are told. Your doctor or endocrinologist may frighten you, if they tell you that your low TSH means you will have a heart attack or stroke, and will have bone loss. You may even go along with a lowering of your dose or even a switch to T4. The results are often disastrous.

I have provided many arguments and pieces of information throughout the book to aid you in convincing your doctor to adopt a more enlightened approach, consistent with recent research findings and facts about how the thyroid hormones actually work.

I am now going to summarise some of the main arguments that may help you, should you need to argue your case. I hope that by putting these in one place here, they may prove powerful should you need to use them.

You may have to be able to argue:

1. Symptoms and signs matter the most. You are collecting these. You need to use them to convince your doctor of what is going on, e.g. that you are not thyrotoxic, or that you are still showing indications of hypothyroidism (regardless of the lab test results).

2. Because T4 is converted within the tissues and T3 is only active within the tissues, hypothyroidism must be diagnosed and treated according to signs and symptoms first, and the FT4 and FT3 levels second.

3. Hypothyroidism is the sub-optimal effect of T3 within the tissues. It is nothing to do with TSH or FT4 levels. Only when the active hormone T3, is at the right level in the tissues (where we cannot measure it), will symptoms resolve.

4. TSH is not a thyroid hormone and its level is not a perfect measure of the body's thyroid status. TSH secretion may be inadequate or dysfunctional for many reasons. TSH cannot be relied upon during treatment as a means of assessing how well the treatment is progressing at all.

5. The thyroid gland puts out T3 when working normally. You deserve to receive some T3 also!

6. T4-Only (T4-monotherapy) may work for some, but almost all studies have shown that it leaves patients with lower FT3 levels than healthy people. T4-Only has been shown in studies to leave persisting hypothyroid symptoms.

7. T4 is not a genuine thyroid hormone; it is relatively inactive. T4 is mainly a prohormone. Your doctor is wrong to assume that the body will always convert it to T3 as needed. There are many reasons why T4 to T3 conversion is poor in some thyroid patients.

8. T4-Only often fails due to poor conversion of T4 to T3, compared to when you were once well. There are many possible reasons for this. A defective DIO1 or DIO2 gene can reduce conversion rate. The loss of thyroid tissue due to Hashimoto's thyroiditis or thyroidectomy will also do this, because the thyroid gland is the most important converter of T4 to T3 in the body. It not only produces some T3, but also converts the T4 contained in the blood that flows through it - like a small, converting machine. Hypocortisolism also impacts thyroid hormone conversion and thyroid effect. Adding T3 to the treatment can help in all of these cases.

9. TSH cannot be used to determine the dose of thyroid replacement, as swallowing T4 or T4/T3 once daily is completely non-physiological. It is not what the TSH-control system was evolved to do. Once on thyroid treatment, your system does not work in the same way that it once did when you were well.

10. Your doctor must treat you firstly according to signs and symptoms, and then secondly according to the FT4 and FT3 levels prior to your first morning thyroid dose.

11. On T4-only, your doctor can increase your dose as needed, guided by symptoms and signs. As long as the FT3 is within-range, your doctor can rest assured that you are not being made thyrotoxic. TSH may fall below the bottom of the reference range, i.e. be suppressed; it is not a concern. See *references 1 and 2* in Resources - you can use these references to persuade your doctor if necessary. These are written by eminent doctors involved in establishing the protocol for hypothyroidism treatment in the UK. They make it very clear that symptom relief is critical and that TSH may or may not be suppressed during treatment. A suppressed TSH is irrelevant if the patient is non-symptomatic and FT3 and FT4 are in range on T4-Only.

12. On T4/T3 or NDT, if the FT4 and FT3 are normal in the morning, prior to your first thyroid medication dose of the day, you cannot be thyrotoxic, as long as you have no signs/symptoms of thyrotoxicity.

13. You may also need to explain how TSH affects the conversion rate of T4 to T3 (see Chapter 4 and Chapter 7), as simply increasing your medication or adding a little T3 to it may not work until TSH is near suppression.

14. Other things can interfere with your treatment. Therefore, getting your doctor to run the right lab tests for nutrients like ferritin, B12, folate and vitamin D is important. Similarly, cortisol may need testing and assessing, given your symptoms. There are significant risks of not assessing cortisol status - see Chapter 5.

15. T3-only therapy is just active hormone therapy and is safe and effective. Signs and symptoms alone must guide it, and the FT3 needs to be high because serum T4 levels are suppressed. See discussion on FT3 reference range in Chapter 14.

16. T3-Only therapy is the treatment of last resort, but it can be extremely effective in resolving symptoms of hypothyroidism. It can also completely get around any conversion issues, or other intracellular problems that stop the other treatments from working well.

I hope these arguments, distilled into one place, are of some use to you. Convincing your doctor of much of the above may be the key to opening the door to better communication with them. If it does not work, you may well have to search for a better doctor.

**Working in partnership with a good doctor**

If you find a doctor that can work with you in partnership, getting well as fast as possible will be within your grasp. I have tried to make you aware of the pitfalls and roadblocks that might be present on this journey. Many of them are there because of current medical practices that are often adhered to robotically. Consequently, I probably seem very negative about doctors during much of this book. I have reason to be from personal experience, and from listening to thousands of thyroid patients who tell me their stories. However, there are good doctors and endocrinologists out there. I know, as I was lucky enough to find some of them eventually. I also know of thyroid patients who have excellent doctors. It can be a good, mutually respectful and productive experience when you find a physician who listens, is highly competent, and wants to work with you to ensure you get healthy and live your life as you deserve to. You just might need to find such a doctor, and work with them in order to get well.

### Getting in the driver's seat

I also urge you to take the above approach *early on*. Please do not squander years of potential good health before you realise that you need to do this. Start as you mean to go on; gain the knowledge that you need and always feel that you own your body and your health and be involved in the process that you need to use to recover. This includes finding the right doctor. It includes working with your doctor and listening to their view. It definitely includes holding on to a different opinion to your doctor if you believe you are right. I would still be ill if I had not done these things.

You will definitely hit roadblocks on the way. Just know that these will happen and that you will have to find a way over, around or through them. Sometimes, you may be able to persuade the person(s) who put them in the way to remove them! There were occasions when I had such setbacks and I started to think that I would just be ill until I died. I did in fact set all my financial affairs in order, assuming that I would probably die before the age of 40. There were times when I was so frustrated that I thought that I would explode! I never gave up totally. Most of the time I just kept going, knowing that I would prevail.

Once in the driver's seat, you can anticipate roadblocks beforehand. You can begin looking into how to get over or through them before you hit them. It will require work on your part to understand and learn the important information (which may well be at odds with current medical practices).

Getting in the driver's seat and being involved in your own health journey can be a really important step towards recovering your health!

### RESOURCES

Here are the two relevant references:

1. ***Thyroid hormone replacement - a counterblast to guidelines*** - Dr A.D. Toft. See: http://www.rcpe.ac.uk/sites/default/files/jrcpe_47_4_toft.pdf
2. ***Consensus statement for good practice and audit measures in the management of hypothyroidism and hyperthyroidism*** - M P J Vanderpump, J A Ahlquist, J A Franklyn, R N Clayton, on behalf of a working group of the Research Unit of the Royal College of Physicians of London, the Endocrinology and Diabetes Committee of the Royal College of Physicians of London, and the Society for Endocrinology See: https://www.ncbi.nlm.nih.gov/pmc/articles/PMC2351923/pdf/bmj00557-0041.pdf

# Chapter 24

# Work, Friends, Family & Children

One of the biggest mistakes that I made, was not anticipating how hard it would be to deal with those around me when I was trying to recover from hypothyroidism.

## WORK

If I had been diagnosed with cancer or a heart problem, this would have been very easy to explain. It would have been easy to tell my boss, colleagues, my family and my small children what was wrong with me, what was likely to happen and how long recovery might take. Moreover, I would have had some idea, during the recovery period, of what I would be able to do and what I would not be capable of doing. People would have understood this.

However, most people do not understand where the thyroid gland is, let alone what it does or how it can turn your life upside down when it does not work properly. If they know anything at all, it will probably be that they know a grandmother or elderly acquaintance that has to take a tablet for their thyroid!

I made so many mistakes in the way I discussed my disease. I should have sat down with my boss, and maybe his boss, my immediate colleagues and Human Resources and explained as much as I could, as simply as possible, about thyroid hormones and how they affect every cell in the body.

If these people had realised that my thyroid hormones were no longer present in sufficient amounts, and even with T4-treatment that they were not working correctly, they might have actually understood what I was going through.

In work, I needed lots of energy to do what I did. It was not a physical job but it was very demanding. I needed to be able to cope with stress. The hypothyroidism that remained, even when on T4-Only, was bad enough. However things were even more difficult with the hypocortisolism that accompanied it. I needed my brain to be in tip-top condition - it was not.

After my initial diagnosis and being given T4-Only, I returned to work. My boss thought I was back to normal, when in fact I was still far from it. He almost immediately gave me two new projects to manage. Even if I had been well, it would have been a huge stretch - maybe even too much for me when I was completely well. I told him that, but it made no difference. I had utterly failed to explain what was going on in my body.

In some jobs, it is risky to suggest that you may not be able to function as you once did. I realise that. You will have to decide for yourself how to handle things.

However, if you *can* be totally open, it might help.

Using the information in Chapters 2 and 4 may enable you to communicate things in a simple and effective way.

I did not get the support that I needed for most of the time during my ill health in work. I say most, because towards the end, I began to pass out due to the hypocortisolism issue that was part of it all. I also lost about 40% of my body weight, so I looked desperately ill. It then became far more obvious to my bosses and colleagues that I was extremely unwell. Eventually, I lost the career that I loved and thrived on. Even if this was not avoidable, it could have been so much less stressful if there had been more support in work.

It is hard enough trying to recover. Trying to recover, in an environment where no one understands what you are going through, is incredibly difficult. Learn from my mistakes!

## FRIENDS

You can use the same approach above with friends. It should be easier. You may need to explain how it is going to affect you. There may be some activities that you feel unable to do right now, or some things that you can attempt, but perhaps not with the same energy that you once had.

Do explain it though. The risk of not doing so is that your friends may think you are just getting depressed or low, or are not interested in them any more. Please avoid all of this. At the point you are trying to recover, you need your friends more than ever.

30 years ago when I was starting to wrestle with hypothyroidism, I did not have the resources that are available now. I had to work it out for myself. I had given up relying on the medical profession to figure out why I did not get well on T4-Only. I had been told too many times, that I would just have to live with it. I had been told too many times, that my symptoms were not to do with hypothyroidism because my labs were within the references ranges! I was still not well, but the doctors just looked at lab results and could not see past them!

I went deep within myself and tried to solve the puzzle. I read second-hand endocrinology books and just kept working on the problem until I understood it and solved it. In the process, I lost contact with many friends. It was a mistake. I should have found a way of balancing things so that I still had my friends and got some support from them. It is, perhaps, part of my nature to focus intensely until I solve something, but I did not get the balance right.

Please do not make the same mistake. It might take some time and effort, but it is worth it.

## FAMILY & CHILDREN

This is probably the biggest area where things can go wrong. It was for me anyway.

I hope most of you who read this book, and perhaps ***Recovering with T3***, or ***The CT3M Handbook,*** get well far more swiftly than I did.

It took me a little over 10 years from diagnosis to recovery. Once I was on an effective dosage of T3, I still had to take things easy, do gentle exercise and build myself back up again. You cannot just bounce straight back when your entire system has been running so poorly for a long time.

In your case, you have a chance to get well quickly and minimise any recovery period. It means that you have the opportunity to limit any damage with relationships within your family, including those with any children.

When you are not the person that you once were, your family, and especially small children, may not understand. Hypothyroidism reduces your energy and enthusiasm, makes you low at times, limits your patience, can affect your mood, can make you cranky and irritable, and will almost certainly make you frustrated. In my case, I was constantly worried about how it would affect my job and how we would cope if I lost it. This was a background worry for the many years during which my hypothyroidism was poorly treated. I may not have discussed this with anyone but it was always in the back of my mind.

Thyroid hormone issues may make you preoccupied with resolving them. This latter point might mean that some amount of your free time may need to go into understanding and resolving the thyroid hormone problem. It might also cost money, as some things need to be done privately.

It can all take its toll at home and with your family. It did for me. I was no longer the same person that I used to be, or the person that I wanted to be.

I will not go into all the consequences for me personally, but they have been very costly indeed, and it has been incredibly painful. I am not unique in this respect. I have heard stories from many thyroid patients who have lost a great deal through this disease and the terribly slow pace of proper diagnosis and proper treatment. These facts, of course, are largely what drove me to write the books, because I know that with proper care and treatment, most of the issues are avoidable.

I am writing this so that you are aware of the possibility that having hypothyroidism, and trying to recover from it, may put a strain on relationships. Explaining things properly and in different ways to adults and children, so that they truly understand what is going on, may help. Being highly aware of how your illness is affecting others will help you to manage things better.

However, the next point is the most important one. ***Getting well as fast as possible is going to be really important. I wrote this book specifically to enable as many people as possible to get well quickly. Achieving this will minimise so many issues.***

I will never be able to put into words how my thyroid issue has changed my life, career and emotional connections with others. I hope that anyone who reads this book has a much smoother journey than I had. Being aware of the potential issues with others may help. Getting well quickly is going to limit any damage. I hope this manual can give you the tools to do this.

# Chapter 25

## Finally - Take Time to Recover & be Kind to Yourself

I believe that all thyroid patients can recover. For some, it may be a short, uneventful journey. For others, it can be an arduous road that requires other problems to be uncovered and resolved along the way.

During this journey, you need to give your body a chance to recover. Putting too many demands on yourself, not asking for help and support, or expecting a 'quick fix' and being disappointed when it does not happen, are not going to help you. You will probably need to adjust your lifestyle to give yourself the best chance of a swift recovery.

If you have been ill for a few years, even when you are on the right treatment and dosage for you, it will still take some time for your body to adjust. It will take time for all the other systems in your body to begin to function as well as they used to do. All the parts of your own energy system have to learn to 'play nicely together' once again.

Starting some gentle exercise can help to stimulate and energise your body and get the mitochondria and adrenals used to working properly again. But exercise only to tolerance and not beyond, or you may pay for it the next day. If there is some activity or sport that you love, trying to do a little of this once more is a good idea. This helped me a lot. Recovery often needs to include both a physical and a psychological aspect. This is especially true if your thyroid hormone issues have gone on for a long time.

Do begin to socialise more if you have stopped doing this. Being with other people is often a boost to the soul, and you need as much of this as possible. Enjoy your family and friends!

You have read this book now. I have put virtually everything that I know, apart from all the details of my T3 protocol, into it. I think I have made it as simple as I can, but I did not dare exclude all the important information that you may need. Some of this information is inherently complex, and no amount of careful writing can make it simple. So, it was a compromise.

The *Thyroid Patient's Manual* can help you on your own journey to good health.
*Please enjoy your time in the driver's seat. Get well and enjoy your life!*

My very best wishes to you all.

*Paul*

# Index

# INDEX

## Q

## R

Rapid heart rate or high heart rate 42, 43, 52, 100, 105, 176

Recording symptoms and signs 103, 109, 111, 112, 115, 116

Reference ranges for a full thyroid panel 60, 108

Reverse T3 (rT3) 24, 25, 26, 31, 32, 34, 39, 44, 51, 52, 59, 60, 61, 63, 65, 97, 98, 107, 108, 124, 125, 126, 132, 133, 134, 135, 140, 141, 144, 146, 152, 153, 154

Root canal infection 91, 176

## S

Selenium 27, 31, 33, 81, 94, 177, 181

Ferritin 27, 78, 79, 81, 94, 175

Serum iron 79, 80, 81

Sex hormones 18, 32, 36, 42, 45, 91, 159, 160, 161, 162, 163, 167, 169, 170, 171

Sex hormone binding globulin (SHBG) 163, 164, 165, 169, 170

Sinus infection *see root canal infection*

Sodium 35, 37, 38, 39, 42, 137, 180

Symptoms of low aldosterone 39, 41, 42, 43, 83, 89

Symptoms of low cortisol 28, 32, 36, 39, 40, 41, 43, 48, 86, 87, 88, 90

Symptoms of low thyroid hormones 29, 62, 63, 98, 105

Synthetic oestradiol 167

Synthroid 118, 121, 129, 183

## T

Testosterone 18, 35, 45, 101, 159, 160, 161, 162, 163, 164, 165, 166, 168, 169, 170, 171, 172

Thyroglobulin (Tg) 23, 30,

Thyroglobulin antibody (TgAb) 30, 59, 60, 61, 62, 108, 110

Thyroid blood tests 25, 43, 57, 59, 64, 65, 107, 124, 133, 144

Thyroid cancer 64, 65, 115

Thyroid enlargement 64

Thyroid forum 67

Thyroid lab test results during treatment 107

Thyroid lab test results when not on any treatment 60

Thyroid nodules 64

Thyroid peroxidase (TPO) 23,

Thyroid peroxidase antibody (TPOAb) 30, 59, 60, 61, 62, 108, 110

Thyroid stimulating hormone (TSH) 19, 20, 21, 23, 27, 29, 30, 32, 33, 34, 44, 51, 52, 53, 55, 56, 59, 60, 61, 62, 63, 64, 65, 66, 101, 107, 108, 109, 110, 111, 114, 115, 121, 122, 123, 124, 1125, 126, 127, 130, 132, 133, 134, 135, 136, 139, 140, 141, 143, 144, 145, 146, 148, 149, 150, 152, 153, 154, 155, 173, 177, 178, 181, 184, 185, 186

Thyroidectomy 27, 32, 110, 141, 183, 185,

Thyrotoxic 108, 109, 125, 138, 139, 185, 186

Thyroxine (T4 or FT4) 9, 20, 23, 24, 25, 26, 27, 28, 29, 31, 32, 33, 34, 39, 51, 52, 53, 55, 56, 59, 60, 61, 62, 63, 64, 65, 67, 71, 77, 78, 95, 102, 103, 104, 107, 108, 109, 110, 111, 112, 113, 114, 115, 117, 118, 119, 121, 122, 123, 124, 125, 126, 127, 129, 130, 132, 133,134, 135, 137, 138, 139, 140, 141, 142, 143, 144, 146, 147, 149, 150, 151, 152, 153, 154, 155, 173, 177, 178, 181, 183, 184, 185, 186, 189, 190

Tiromel 137

Total iron binding capacity (TIBC) 79, 80, 81

Toxicity 131, 175, 176

Triiodothyronine (T3 or FT3) 9, 20, 23, 24, 25, 26, 27, 28, 29, 31, 32, 33, 34, 39, 43, 44, 48, 51, 52, 53, 54, 55, 56, 59, 60, 61, 62, 63, 64, 65, 66, 67, 69, 71, 77, 78, 84, 89, 90, 91, 92, 95, 97, 98, 101, 102, 103, 104, 105, 107, 108, 109, 110, 111, 112, 113, 114, 115, 116, 117, 118, 119, 121, 122, 123, 124, 125, 126, 127, 129, 130, 131, 132, 134, 135, 136, 137, 138, 139, 140, 141, 142, 143, 144, 145, 146, 147, 148, 149, 150, 151, 152, 153, 154, 155, 173, 176, 177, 178, 181, 183, 184, 185, 186, 190, 193

Transferrin or transferrin saturation % 79, 80, 81

T1 or T2 24, 26, 129, 137

T3 half-life 140,

T3 is far more potent than T4 137

T3-monotherapy, *see T3-Only*

T3-Only treatment 52, 112, 113, 134, 137, 144, 148, 149

T4 half-life 122, 124, 130, 141, 150

T4-monotherapy, *see T4-Only*

T4-Only treatment 103, 121, 123, 125, 127, 149

T4 to T3 conversion or conversion (of T4 to T3) 23, 24, 25, 26, 27, 28, 31, 32, 33, 34, 39, 51, 52, 53, 56, 61, 63, 71, 77, 78, 95, 109, 110, 111, 112, 113, 116, 122, 123, 124, 125, 130, 133, 134, 137, 138, 140, 141, 142, 150, 152, 153, 178, 181, 183, 185, 186

T4/T3 treatment 149, 150, 151, 152, 153, 154, 155

## U

Uterus 19, 161, 167

Uterine cancer or uterine cancer risk167

## V

Vitamin A 173, 181

Vitamin B3 or B3 48, 94

Vitamin B12 71, 72, 73, 74, 75, 82, 94, 99, 146, 173, 178, 179

Vitamin B complex 94, 162

Vitamin C 79, 81, 93, 94, 95, 162